For Paris Neil

Table of Contents:

Introduction:
- Understanding Anxiety: A Personal Journey
- The Importance of Seeking Help

Chapter 1: What Are Anxiety Disorders? P.7
- Defining Generalized Anxiety Disorder (GAD)
- Understanding Panic Disorder
- Common Symptoms and Triggers

Chapter 2: The Science Behind Anxiety P.20
- How Anxiety Affects the Brain
- The Role of Genetics and Environment
- Understanding the Stress Response

Chapter 3: Recognizing Your Anxiety P.32
- Identifying Your Triggers
- The Importance of Self-Awareness
- Keeping a Journal: Tracking Your Thoughts and Feelings
- Subjective Units of Distress (SUD) Scale
- Narrative Therapy and Self-Awareness

Chapter 4: Coping Strategies and Techniques P.57
- Breathing Exercises for Immediate Relief
- Mindfulness and Meditation Practices

- Grounding Techniques for Panic Attacks
- Progressive Muscle Relaxation (PMR)

<u>Chapter 5: Cognitive Behavioral Therapy (CBT) P.84</u>
- Understanding CBT and Its Benefits
- Challenging Negative Thoughts using CBT
- Practical CBT Exercises

<u>Chapter 6: Positive Psychology for Anxiety P.104</u>
- Understanding Positive Psychology and Its Benefits
- Challenging Negative Thoughts using Positive Psychology
- Positive Emotion, Engagement, Relationships, Meaning, and Accomplishment
  (PERMA)

<u>Chapter 7: Mindfulness Based Stress Reduction (MBSR) P.126</u>
- Understanding MBSR and Its Benefits
- Challenging Negative Thoughts using MBSR

<u>Chapter 8: Lifestyle Changes for Better Mental Health P.137</u>
- Nutrition and Its Impact on Anxiety
- The Role of Exercise in Reducing Anxiety
- Sleep Hygiene: Importance of Rest
- Music Therapy

Chapter 9: Building a Support System P.158

- The Importance of Communication
- Finding Support Groups
- Involving Family and Friends in Your Journey
- Animal- assisted therapy

Chapter 10: When to Seek Professional Help P.198
- Different Types of Therapists and Treatments
- Medication Options for Anxiety Disorders
- What to Expect in Therapy

Chapter 11: Long-Term Strategies P.223
- Developing a Personal Action Plan
- Maintaining Progress and Celebrating Success
- Lessons Learned and Hope for the Future
- Embracing Life Beyond Anxiety
- Final Thoughts and Encouragement

My journey with anxiety began over 20 years ago on Broad Street in South Philadelphia, where I ironically experienced my very first panic attack while attending a positive psychology summit at the University of Pennsylvania. At that moment, I had no idea what was happening to me. The overwhelming sense of dread and the physical sensations of panic were foreign and terrifying. This experience marked the start of a long and arduous journey that would change my life forever. In the years that followed, I faced the daunting challenge of enduring over 10,000 panic attacks. Each one felt like an insurmountable wave crashing over me, leaving me gasping for breath and grasping for control. The relentless cycle of anxiety led to significant avoidance behaviors; I withdrew from social situations, turned down career opportunities, and constantly lived in fear of the next attack. My life became a series of carefully orchestrated plans to avoid triggers, which only deepened my sense of isolation and despair. But amidst the turmoil, I was determined to find a way out.

Realizing that nothing ever really happened after these panic attacks, I started to figure out multiple theories and coping skills that would help me reduce each panic attack thereafter. I immersed myself in research, seeking to understand the mechanisms behind anxiety and panic. I explored various therapeutic approaches, experimented with mindfulness techniques, and developed my own strategies for cultivating a calm mindset. Over time, I learned through continuous research in the field of psychology, particularly Mindful Based Stress Reduction and Positive Psychology that I could face my fears rather than flee from them. I discovered that even under pressure, I had the capacity to remain calm and centered. My experiences have shaped me into a passionate advocate for mental health. Now, as an author and speaker, I share my story and the strategies I've developed to help others reclaim their lives from anxiety. I believe that everyone has the potential to find peace, even in the midst of chaos. Through my work, I aim to inspire others to confront their fears and embrace a life filled with hope and possibility. Together, we can break free from the constraints of anxiety and find the calm we all deserve.

This book aims to provide a comprehensive guide for individuals struggling with generalized anxiety disorder and panic disorder, offering practical tools, personal stories, and strategies to foster resilience and healing.

Chapter 1: What Are Anxiety Disorders?

Understanding Anxiety: A Personal Journey - My introspective journey has sparked the development of a specific set of theories and strategies that, over time, started to make a profound difference in my life. These theories were rooted in understanding the interplay between thoughts, emotions, and bodily sensations. I learned to identify the triggers that set off my panic attacks and developed practical tools to manage my reactions. I began to focus on cultivating a mindset that embraced calmness, even in the face of fear. This approach not only transformed my own experience but also resonated with many others in my network who were grappling with similar challenges.

As I shared my insights and strategies with friends, family, and support groups, I was amazed to see how these concepts could help others reclaim their lives from the grips of anxiety. It became clear that the techniques I developed were not just beneficial for me but had the potential to affect thousands of lives. My personal journey has taught me that while the road to recovery may be long and fraught with challenges, it is possible to find a path to peace. I stand as a testament to the power of perseverance and the potential for healing when we are willing to explore alternative approaches. Anxiety may be a part of my story, but it does not define me. Through understanding and sharing what I have learned, I hope to empower others to navigate their own journeys with courage and resilience.

In the journey of managing anxiety, one of the most crucial steps is recognizing the importance of seeking help. It can be incredibly daunting to admit that we need support, especially when we feel trapped in our own minds. However, reaching out for assistance is not a sign of weakness; rather, it is an empowering decision that can lead to profound transformation.

Below, you will find a list of steps that can empower you to seek help whenever needed.

1. Breaking the Isolation: Anxiety disorders often come with a heavy burden of isolation. Many individuals feel alone in their struggles, believing that no one understands what they are going through. Seeking help allows us to break this cycle of solitude. Whether through therapy, support groups, or simply confiding in trusted friends or family members, sharing our experiences can alleviate the sense of isolation and foster a sense of community.

2. Accessing Professional Expertise: Mental health professionals possess the training, experience, and tools to help navigate the complexities of anxiety. They can provide tailored strategies and coping mechanisms that we may not have considered. Professional guidance can be instrumental

in helping us understand our thoughts and behaviors, uncover underlying issues, and develop effective treatment plans.

3. Identifying and Understanding Triggers: One of the challenges of anxiety is recognizing the specific triggers that provoke our symptoms. A mental health professional can help us identify these triggers and provide insight into how they impact our daily lives. This understanding is vital for developing proactive strategies to manage anxiety and reduce the frequency and intensity of panic attacks.

4. Encouraging Accountability: Seeking help creates a support system that holds us accountable for our healing journey. Regular check-ins with a therapist or participation in support groups can motivate us to stay committed to our goals and practice the techniques we learn. This accountability can be a powerful catalyst for positive change.

5. Exploring Treatment Options: There is no one-size-fits-all solution for anxiety disorders. By seeking help, we open ourselves up to a variety of treatment modalities, including therapy, medication, lifestyle changes, and mindfulness practices. A mental health professional can guide us through these options, helping us find the right combination that works for our unique needs.

6. Fostering Personal Growth: Engaging in therapy or support groups often leads to personal growth and self-discovery. As

we confront our fears and learn more about ourselves, we develop resilience and coping skills that extend beyond anxiety. This journey can foster a deeper understanding of our emotions, enhance our relationships, and empower us to face life's challenges with greater confidence.

7. Normalizing the Experience: Lastly, seeking help helps to normalize the conversation around mental health. By talking openly about our struggles, we contribute to breaking the stigma associated with anxiety disorders. This, in turn, encourages others to seek help as well, creating a culture of understanding and support. In conclusion, seeking help is a vital step in the journey of overcoming anxiety. It allows us to break free from isolation, access professional guidance, and develop the skills necessary to manage our symptoms effectively.

By reaching out, we take a courageous step toward healing, personal growth, and ultimately, a more fulfilling life. Remember, you are not alone in this journey, and there is strength in seeking the help you deserve.

The DSM-5, or the Diagnostic and Statistical Manual of Mental Disorders, Fifth Edition, is a comprehensive classification system published by the American Psychiatric Association (APA) used by mental health professionals to diagnose and classify mental disorders. It serves as a critical tool for clinicians, researchers, and educators in the field of psychology and psychiatry.

Key Features of the DSM-5: *1. Diagnostic Criteria: The DSM-5 provides specific criteria that must be met for a diagnosis of various mental disorders. Each disorder is described in detail, including its symptoms, duration, and severity.*

2. Classification System: The manual categorizes mental disorders into various groups based on shared characteristics. For example, it includes mood disorders, anxiety disorders, psychotic disorders, and personality disorders, among others.

3. Descriptive Text: Alongside the diagnostic criteria, the DSM-5 includes descriptive text that provides context, prevalence rates, risk factors, and cultural considerations related to each disorder.

4. Cultural Sensitivity: The DSM-5 emphasizes the importance of cultural factors in diagnosis and recognizes that cultural differences can influence the presentation and interpretation of mental health symptoms.

5. Research and Updates: The DSM-5 is regularly updated to reflect new research findings and changes in the understanding of mental health conditions. This ensures that the diagnostic criteria remain relevant and evidence-based.

6. Use in Treatment Planning: While primarily a diagnostic tool, the DSM-5 also aids in treatment planning by providing information on commonly used interventions for specific disorders.

7. International Use: While the DSM-5 is primarily used in the United States, it has also gained international recognition and is often used in research and clinical practice worldwide. The DSM-5 is essential for standardizing the diagnosis of mental health disorders, facilitating communication among professionals, and guiding research and treatment approaches in the field of mental health.

Generalized Anxiety Disorder (GAD) is classified in the Diagnostic and Statistical Manual of Mental Disorders, Fifth Edition (DSM-5), as a condition characterized by excessive and uncontrollable worry about various aspects of life, which can lead to significant distress and impairment in functioning.

Key Features of GAD According to DSM-5:

1. Excessive Worry: Individuals with GAD experience persistent and excessive worry about multiple events or activities, such as work, health, or social interactions. This worry occurs more days than not for at least six months.

2. Difficulty Controlling Worry: The worry is difficult for the individual to control, often leading to a cycle of anxiety that can be overwhelming.

3. Associated Symptoms: In addition to excessive worry, GAD is associated with several physical and psychological symptoms, including: - Restlessness or feeling keyed up or on edge - Easily fatigued - Difficulty concentrating or mind going blank - Irritability - Muscle tension - Sleep disturbances (difficulty falling asleep, staying asleep, or restless sleep)

4. Impact on Functioning: The anxiety and worry must cause clinically significant distress or impairment in social, occupational, or other important areas of functioning.

5. Exclusion of Other Disorders: The symptoms must not be attributable to the physiological effects of a substance or another medical condition, and the worry should not be better explained by another mental disorder.

Treatment Options: The DSM-5 also acknowledges various treatment options for GAD, which may include psychotherapy (such as cognitive-behavioral therapy), medication (like SSRIs or SNRIs), or a combination of both. The focus of treatment is on helping individuals manage their anxiety and improve their quality of life. Overall, GAD is a common and often debilitating condition that requires appropriate assessment and intervention to help individuals regain control over their anxiety and enhance their daily functioning.

"What Are Anxiety Disorders?", typically provides an overview of anxiety disorders, defining what they are and how they manifest in individuals. It explains that anxiety disorders are a group of mental health conditions characterized by excessive fear or worry that can interfere with daily activities. The chapter often outlines the different types of anxiety disorders, including generalized anxiety disorder (GAD), panic disorder, social anxiety disorder, and specific phobias, highlighting their unique symptoms and impacts on individuals.

It may also discuss the prevalence of these disorders, noting how common they are in various populations. Furthermore, the chapter usually touches on the physiological and psychological aspects of anxiety, explaining how anxiety can trigger a fight-or-flight response and the role of neurotransmitters in this process. It may also introduce the concept of risk factors, including genetics, environment, and personal history, that contribute to the development of anxiety disorders. Overall, this chapter serves as a foundational introduction to understanding anxiety disorders, setting the stage for deeper exploration of their causes, symptoms, and treatment options in subsequent chapters.

Understanding Panic Disorder Panic Disorder is a type of anxiety disorder characterized by recurrent and unexpected panic attacks, which are sudden periods of intense fear or discomfort that peak within minutes. Individuals with panic disorder often live in fear of experiencing future attacks, which can lead to significant avoidance behaviors and impact daily functioning.

Panic Attacks: These are the hallmark of panic disorder. A panic attack typically includes a variety of physical and emotional symptoms that can be overwhelming.

Fear of Future Attacks: Many individuals develop a persistent worry about having more attacks, which can influence their behavior and lead to avoidance of certain situations or places.
-

Avoidance Behavior: To prevent the possibility of a panic attack, individuals may avoid places where they previously experienced an attack or situations they perceive as anxiety-inducing (e.g., crowded places, public transportation).

Common Symptoms and Triggers

Common Symptoms: Panic attacks can manifest through a variety of physical and psychological symptoms, including:

Physical Symptoms: - Rapid heart rate (palpitations) - Shortness of breath or difficulty breathing - Chest pain or discomfort - Sweating - Trembling or shaking - Dizziness, lightheadedness, or feeling faint - Nausea or abdominal distress - Chills or hot flashes - Numbness or tingling sensations - Psychological Symptoms: - Feelings of unreality or detachment from oneself (derealization or depersonalization) - Fear of losing control or "going crazy" - Fear of dying

Common Triggers: The triggers for panic attacks can vary widely from person to person, but some common triggers include: - Stressful Life Events:Major changes, such as the death of a loved one, divorce, or job loss, can trigger panic attacks.

Health Concerns: Worrying about health issues or experiencing physical symptoms can lead to panic attacks. - Certain Situations: Enclosed spaces (like elevators), crowded areas, or situations where escape might be difficult can trigger anxiety and lead to panic attacks.

Substance Use:*Caffeine, alcohol, or certain drugs can increase anxiety and trigger panic attacks.

Past Experiences: Previous panic attacks can create a fear of similar situations, leading to conditioned responses. Understanding panic disorder and its symptoms can help individuals identify their experiences and seek appropriate treatment, which may include therapy, medication, or lifestyle changes to manage anxiety and reduce the frequency of panic attacks.

Triggers for panic disorder can be complex and vary significantly between individuals. Understanding these triggers is crucial for managing and reducing the occurrence of panic attacks.

Here are some common categories of triggers, along with specific examples:

Environmental Triggers - These are external situations or settings that can provoke anxiety and lead to panic attacks. - Crowded Places: Being in a busy shopping mall, concert, or public transport can induce feelings of being trapped or overwhelmed. - Enclosed Spaces: Elevators, small rooms, or airplanes can trigger feelings of claustrophobia. - Unfamiliar Locations:New or unfamiliar environments can heighten anxiety and lead to panic.

Emotional Triggers - Certain emotional states or experiences can act as triggers for panic attacks. - Stress:High levels of stress from work, relationships, or financial issues can increase anxiety levels. - Negative Emotions: Feelings of sadness, anger, or frustration can lead to panic attacks, especially if the individual feels unable to express or manage these emotions. - Anticipation of Stressful Events: Worrying about upcoming events, such as public speaking or important meetings, can trigger panic.

<u>Physical Triggers</u> - Physical sensations or conditions can also provoke panic attacks. - Body Sensations: Experiencing physical symptoms such as rapid heartbeat, dizziness, or shortness of breath can create a fear of having a panic attack, leading to a self-perpetuating cycle. - Fatigue: Lack of sleep or physical exhaustion can heighten anxiety levels and make panic attacks more likely. - Health Issues: Chronic illnesses or sudden health scares (e.g., chest pain) can trigger panic due to fear of serious medical conditions.

<u>Substance Related Triggers</u> - The use of certain substances can increase the likelihood of panic attacks. - Caffeine: High intake of caffeine can lead to increased heart rate and anxiety, which may trigger panic attacks. - Alcohol: While some may use alcohol to self-medicate anxiety, withdrawal or overconsumption can lead to increased anxiety and panic. - Recreational Drugs:Stimulants or drugs that affect mood can provoke panic attacks, especially in individuals predisposed to anxiety disorders.

<u>Social Triggers</u> - Social situations can be particularly challenging for those with panic disorder. - Social Interactions: Large gatherings, parties, or even meeting new people can

lead to anxiety and panic. - Performance Situations: Activities that require public speaking, performing, or being the center of attention can be triggering.

<u>Cognitive Triggers</u> - Thought patterns and beliefs can also act as triggers. - Catastrophic Thinking: The tendency to interpret physical sensations or everyday stressors as signs of impending doom can lead to panic. - Fear of Losing Control: Worrying about losing control in social situations or during a panic attack itself can trigger further anxiety.

Coping and Management Identifying personal triggers is an essential step in managing panic disorder. Keeping a journal to track when panic attacks occur and what preceded them can help individuals recognize patterns. Strategies such as cognitive-behavioral therapy (CBT), mindfulness practices, and relaxation techniques can also aid in managing triggers and reducing the frequency of panic attacks.

By understanding and addressing these triggers, individuals can take proactive steps toward managing their panic disorder and improving their overall quality of life.

Chapter 2: The Science Behind Anxiety

Anxiety is an intricate part of the human experience, rooted deeply in our biology and psychology. At its core, anxiety is not just an emotional reaction; it is a complex interplay of neural pathways, hormonal responses, and cognitive processes designed to protect us from harm. While it can be adaptive in helping us respond to threats, anxiety becomes problematic when it spirals out of control, manifesting as overwhelming fear, avoidance, and physiological distress.

In this chapter, we will unravel the science behind anxiety—exploring how our brains and bodies are wired to perceive danger, how these mechanisms have evolved over time, and why they sometimes misfire. We'll take a closer look at the role of key brain structures like the amygdala and prefrontal cortex, and how neurotransmitters like serotonin, dopamine, and GABA influence anxious responses.

Understanding the biological and psychological underpinnings of anxiety is crucial for two reasons. First, it demystifies the condition, providing insight into why we feel the way we do during moments of heightened stress or fear. Second, it lays the groundwork for developing effective strategies to manage and overcome anxiety, whether through therapy, medication, lifestyle changes, or a combination of approaches.

By delving into the science, this chapter seeks to provide clarity and empowerment—equipping you with knowledge that transforms anxiety from an overwhelming mystery into a challenge that can be understood and addressed. Let's explore the fascinating mechanisms that drive this universal human experience and uncover the keys to taking control of it.

How Anxiety Affects the Brain

Anxiety has profound effects on the brain, shaping how we process information, perceive threats, and react to the world around us. It engages specific neural circuits, triggering a cascade of responses designed to protect us. However, when anxiety becomes chronic or exaggerated, these responses can disrupt normal functioning, creating a vicious cycle of fear and stress.

The Amygdala: The Alarm System

The amygdala, an almond-shaped structure deep within the brain, plays a central role in anxiety. Often referred to as the brain's "alarm system," the amygdala detects potential threats and initiates a fight-or-flight response. When the amygdala is overactive, it can perceive danger where none exists, leading to heightened vigilance, fear, and avoidance behaviors.

The Prefrontal Cortex: The Voice of Reason

The prefrontal cortex, located at the front of the brain, helps regulate emotional responses and assess the reality of perceived threats. In individuals with anxiety, the connection between the prefrontal cortex and the amygdala is often weakened, making it harder to override irrational fears with logical reasoning. This imbalance can lead to an inability to calm down even when a situation is objectively safe.

The Role of Neurotransmitters

Chemical messengers in the brain, known as neurotransmitters, play a vital role in regulating mood and anxiety. Key players include:

- **Serotonin**: Often referred to as the "feel-good" neurotransmitter, low levels of serotonin are associated with increased anxiety.
- **Gamma-Aminobutyric Acid (GABA)**: This inhibitory neurotransmitter helps calm brain activity. A deficiency in GABA can result in heightened excitability and anxiety.
- **Dopamine**: Involved in reward and motivation, dopamine imbalances can exacerbate feelings of anxiety, particularly when linked to social situations.

The Hypothalamic-Pituitary-Adrenal (HPA) Axis: The Stress Regulator

The HPA axis governs the body's response to stress by releasing cortisol, a hormone that helps prepare the body for action. In individuals with chronic anxiety, the HPA axis can become dysregulated, leading to prolonged cortisol release. This not only affects the brain but also impacts the body, contributing to fatigue, weakened immune function, and difficulty concentrating.

Neuroplasticity and Anxiety

Interestingly, the brain's ability to adapt—known as neuroplasticity—also plays a role in anxiety. Chronic anxiety can strengthen neural pathways associated with fear and worry, making it harder to break free from anxious thought patterns. However, the same plasticity offers hope: with the right interventions, such as cognitive-behavioral therapy (CBT) or mindfulness practices, these pathways can be rewired, creating new patterns of calm and resilience.

Understanding how anxiety affects the brain provides a foundation for managing it. By addressing the overactive amygdala, strengthening the prefrontal cortex's regulatory abilities, and rebalancing neurotransmitters, it's possible to regain control and restore mental harmony. In the next section, we'll explore how anxiety's effects on the brain manifest in the body and everyday life, bringing the science into sharper focus.

The Role of Genetics and Environment

Anxiety doesn't arise in isolation. It is shaped by a combination of genetic predispositions and environmental influences, which interact in complex ways to determine how an individual experiences and responds to stress. While some people may inherit a heightened sensitivity to anxiety, life experiences and environmental factors play a critical role in amplifying or mitigating that predisposition.

Genetics: The Blueprint for Vulnerability

Research has shown that anxiety disorders often run in families, suggesting a genetic component. Specific genes influence the way the brain processes stress and fear, particularly those involved in the production and regulation of neurotransmitters like serotonin and GABA. For instance:

- **Serotonin Transporter Gene (SLC6A4)**: Variations in this gene can affect serotonin levels, making individuals more prone to anxiety and depression.
- **COMT Gene**: This gene regulates dopamine in the prefrontal cortex. Variants associated with slower dopamine breakdown may lead to heightened sensitivity to stress.

While genetics can increase susceptibility to anxiety, they do not guarantee its development. Genes interact with life experiences, meaning that environmental factors often determine whether or not someone with a genetic predisposition will develop an anxiety disorder.

The Environment: Shaping the Experience

The environment plays a crucial role in triggering or exacerbating anxiety. Key environmental factors include:

- **Early Childhood Experiences**: Adverse childhood experiences (ACEs), such as abuse, neglect, or

exposure to parental conflict, can sensitize the brain's fear response system, leading to an increased risk of anxiety in adulthood.
- **Trauma and Stress**: Significant life events, such as accidents, loss of a loved one, or financial instability, can activate or worsen anxiety, particularly in individuals with a genetic predisposition.
- **Parenting Styles**: Overprotective or overly critical parenting can increase a child's likelihood of developing anxiety by reinforcing fears and limiting opportunities for resilience-building.
- **Cultural and Social Influences**: Living in a high-stress environment, experiencing discrimination, or being exposed to societal pressures can contribute to chronic anxiety.

Gene-Environment Interaction

The interplay between genetics and the environment is a dynamic process. For instance, someone with a genetic predisposition for anxiety might never develop symptoms if they grow up in a nurturing, supportive environment. Conversely, environmental stressors may "activate" genetic vulnerabilities, leading to heightened anxiety responses.

One striking example of this interplay is epigenetics—the process by which environmental factors influence gene expression. Stressful or traumatic events can cause certain genes to become more active, potentially increasing anxiety. These changes can sometimes even be passed onto future generations, further illustrating the complex relationship between genes and environment.

Resilience: Overcoming Genetic and Environmental Challenges

It's important to note that neither genetics nor environment determines an individual's fate. Resilience-building factors, such as supportive relationships, positive coping mechanisms, and access to therapy or medication, can mitigate both genetic and environmental risks. Practices like mindfulness, regular exercise, and developing a growth mindset can help reshape how the brain and body respond to anxiety-inducing situations.

By understanding the intricate roles of genetics and environment in anxiety, we can better appreciate its multifaceted nature. This awareness allows for more personalized approaches to treatment, focusing on not only the biological and psychological aspects but also the contextual factors that shape each individual's experience.

In the next section, we'll examine how anxiety manifests in the body, exploring the physical symptoms and their connection to the brain's activity.

Understanding the Stress Response

The stress response is an ancient survival mechanism designed to help us react quickly to threats, ensuring our safety and survival. While it's highly effective in short-term situations—like escaping a predator or avoiding danger—it can become problematic when triggered too often or inappropriately, as is often the case with anxiety.

The Brain's Role in the Stress Response

The stress response begins in the brain, specifically in the **amygdala**, which acts as a sentinel, scanning for potential threats. If the amygdala detects danger, it sends a distress signal to the **hypothalamus**, the brain's control center for bodily functions.

From here, two major systems are activated:

1. **Sympathetic Nervous System (SNS)**: The SNS immediately prepares the body to respond to danger. This system triggers a cascade of changes to optimize physical and mental readiness:
    - **Heart Rate and Blood Pressure Spike**: Blood is redirected to muscles, enabling rapid movement.
    - **Breathing Quickens**: To increase oxygen intake for energy production.
    - **Energy Stores Are Released**: Glucose and fatty acids flood the bloodstream, providing the body with immediate fuel.

- ○ **Heightened Senses**: Vision sharpens, hearing becomes more acute, and focus narrows to the perceived threat.
2. **Hypothalamic-Pituitary-Adrenal (HPA) Axis**: This slower but equally important system involves the release of **cortisol**, the primary stress hormone. Cortisol sustains energy levels and keeps the body on high alert.

These responses are essential in life-or-death situations, but when they are frequently activated in response to non-life-threatening stressors—such as work deadlines or social anxiety—they can cause physical and psychological strain.

The Physical Effects of Chronic Stress

When the stress response becomes chronic, it disrupts the body's equilibrium. Instead of activating only in response to genuine threats, the body stays in a heightened state of vigilance, leading to:

- **Cardiovascular Strain**: Persistent high blood pressure and heart rate increase the risk of heart disease and stroke.
- **Respiratory Issues**: Chronic rapid breathing can lead to hyperventilation and shortness of breath, common in anxiety disorders.
- **Digestive Problems**: Stress suppresses digestion, which can result in stomach pain, nausea, or irritable bowel syndrome (IBS).

- **Immune Suppression**: Elevated cortisol levels weaken the immune system, making the body more susceptible to infections.
- **Muscle Tension**: Prolonged activation of the SNS causes chronic tension, leading to headaches, jaw pain, and other physical discomforts.

The Mental and Emotional Impact

Chronic stress doesn't only affect the body; it also takes a significant toll on the brain and emotional well-being:

- **Overactive Amygdala**: Chronic stress strengthens neural connections in the amygdala, making the brain more sensitive to perceived threats.
- **Weakened Prefrontal Cortex**: The prefrontal cortex, responsible for rational thinking and decision-making, becomes less effective in regulating emotional responses, exacerbating feelings of worry and fear.
- **Memory and Focus Issues**: Excess cortisol impairs the hippocampus, the brain's memory center, leading to forgetfulness and difficulty concentrating.
- **Mood Dysregulation**: Chronic stress can lead to irritability, sadness, and a sense of overwhelm, laying the groundwork for anxiety disorders and depression.

Anxiety and the Hijacked Stress Response

For individuals with anxiety, the stress response can become "hijacked." This means that the brain begins to react to benign situations—like speaking in public or being in a crowded room—as if they were life-threatening. This misfiring creates a cycle:

1. A harmless trigger activates the stress response.
2. The physical sensations of stress (e.g., rapid heartbeat, sweating) reinforce the perception of danger.
3. The brain learns to associate the trigger with anxiety, making future encounters even more distressing.

Over time, this cycle can lead to avoidance behaviors and heightened sensitivity to stress, further entrenching anxiety.

Restoring Balance to the Stress Response

Breaking the cycle of chronic stress requires retraining the brain and body to respond appropriately to threats. Techniques that can help include:

- **Mindfulness and Relaxation Practices**: Meditation, deep breathing, and yoga activate the parasympathetic nervous system (PNS), counteracting the stress response.
- **Cognitive-Behavioral Therapy (CBT)**: CBT helps identify and challenge irrational fears, reducing the frequency and intensity of the stress response.
- **Physical Activity**: Exercise reduces cortisol levels and promotes the release of endorphins, the body's natural stress relievers.
- **Adequate Rest and Nutrition**: Sleep and a balanced diet support the body's ability to regulate cortisol and maintain equilibrium.

By understanding the science of the stress response, we can better recognize its role in anxiety and take deliberate steps to regain control. In the next section, we'll explore practical strategies to disrupt the anxiety cycle and promote long-term resilience.

Chapter 3: Recognizing Your Anxiety

The first step to managing anxiety is recognizing it. While anxiety is a natural response to stress, it can manifest in ways that are subtle, complex, and sometimes confusing. Understanding the signs and symptoms of anxiety, and how they uniquely show up in your life, is crucial for gaining control over it.

Anxiety doesn't look the same for everyone. It can be a constant feeling of unease, a sudden surge of panic, or even physical symptoms like muscle tension or headaches. For some, it's a quiet whisper of doubt that colors everyday interactions. For others, it's a loud and overwhelming voice that dominates their thoughts. Recognizing your anxiety means identifying these patterns, understanding their triggers, and learning how they impact your daily life.

The Physical Symptoms of Anxiety

Anxiety often begins in the mind but quickly makes itself known in the body. Common physical symptoms include:

- **Racing Heartbeat**: The sensation of your heart pounding as adrenaline courses through your system.
- **Shortness of Breath**: Difficulty breathing or feeling as though you can't get enough air.
- **Muscle Tension**: Tightness in the shoulders, neck, or jaw that persists even in the absence of obvious stress.

- **Stomach Problems**: Nausea, indigestion, or a feeling of butterflies in the stomach.
- **Sweating or Shaking**: Uncontrollable physical reactions to fear or stress.
- **Fatigue or Insomnia**: Anxiety can leave you feeling drained, or it may keep you awake with racing thoughts.

These physical sensations are part of the body's fight-or-flight response, often triggered unnecessarily by anxiety disorders. Recognizing these signs is key to understanding how anxiety affects you.

The Emotional Symptoms of Anxiety

Anxiety can also affect how you feel emotionally, creating a mental landscape dominated by fear and worry. Emotional symptoms include:

- **Irrational Worries**: Persistent fears that may seem out of proportion to the actual situation.
- **Restlessness**: Feeling "on edge" or unable to relax.
- **Irritability**: Small frustrations can seem overwhelming, leading to anger or annoyance.
- **Overthinking**: Replaying past events or imagining worst-case scenarios in the future.
- **Difficulty Focusing**: Feeling distracted or unable to concentrate due to intrusive thoughts.

Anxiety doesn't just stay in your head; it influences how you act. Recognizing behavior changes can help pinpoint how anxiety is shaping your life. Common patterns include:

- **Avoidance**: Steering clear of situations, places, or people that might trigger anxiety.
- **Compulsive Behaviors**: Repeating certain actions (like checking locks or seeking reassurance) to soothe anxious thoughts.
- **Procrastination**: Delaying tasks out of fear of failure or judgment.
- **Social Withdrawal**: Isolating yourself from others due to feelings of insecurity or overwhelm.

Identifying Your Triggers

Anxiety is often triggered by specific situations, thoughts, or experiences. These triggers can be obvious, like speaking in public or meeting a deadline, or subtle, like certain sounds, smells, or memories. Keeping a journal to track when your anxiety occurs can help you identify patterns and gain insight into your personal triggers.

Accepting Your Anxiety

Recognizing your anxiety isn't just about identifying symptoms—it's also about accepting them without judgment. Anxiety is a natural human experience, and acknowledging its presence is the first step toward managing it. By treating your anxiety as a signal rather than a flaw, you can begin to approach it with curiosity and compassion.

In this chapter, we'll delve deeper into the various types of anxiety, helping you pinpoint whether your experience aligns with generalized anxiety, social anxiety, panic disorder, or another condition. Armed with this understanding, you'll be better prepared to address your anxiety and take steps toward overcoming it.

How to Identify Your Triggers

Identifying your anxiety triggers is a powerful step toward understanding and managing your emotions. Triggers are the events, situations, thoughts, or sensations that initiate feelings of anxiety. While some triggers are obvious, others can be subtle or deeply rooted in past experiences. By uncovering your triggers, you can take steps to manage your reactions and reduce the power they hold over you.

The Different Types of Triggers

1. **External Triggers**: These are events or situations in your environment that provoke anxiety. Examples include:
    - Deadlines or high-pressure work environments.
    - Public speaking or social interactions.
    - Conflicts with family, friends, or coworkers.
    - Financial difficulties.

- Certain places, like crowded areas or unfamiliar settings.
2. **Internal Triggers**: These originate from within and may be linked to thoughts, memories, or physical sensations. Examples include:
    - Self-critical or perfectionistic thoughts.
    - Flashbacks to past trauma.
    - Feeling lightheaded, short of breath, or experiencing other bodily sensations that mimic anxiety.
3. **Subtle Triggers**: These are less obvious and often harder to identify, but they can significantly impact your anxiety levels. Examples include:
    - Certain smells, sounds, or colors associated with negative memories.
    - News headlines or stories that remind you of personal fears.
    - Changes in routine, even minor ones.

Steps to Identify Your Triggers

1. **Keep an Anxiety Journal**

   Tracking your experiences can help you uncover patterns and pinpoint triggers. Each time you feel anxious, write down:
    - What was happening before your anxiety began.
    - Your thoughts, emotions, and physical sensations.
    - The intensity of your anxiety on a scale of 1 to 10.

2. Over time, recurring themes will emerge, helping you identify the causes of your anxiety.
3. **Reflect on Past Experiences**
Anxiety triggers are often rooted in past experiences. Reflect on situations where you felt anxious and ask yourself:
    - What was happening at the time?
    - Were there similarities to other anxiety-inducing situations?
    - Could this be linked to an earlier traumatic or stressful event?
4. **Pay Attention to Your Body**
Your body often reacts to triggers before your mind recognizes them. Notice patterns in your physical responses, such as:
    - Tension in your shoulders or jaw.
    - A racing heartbeat or sweaty palms.
    - Restlessness or a sudden urge to leave a situation.
5. These physical cues can provide valuable insight into your anxiety triggers.
6. **Examine Your Thoughts**
Anxiety often stems from thought patterns that amplify fear. When you feel anxious, ask yourself:
    - What am I thinking about right now?
    - Am I imagining a worst-case scenario?
    - Is this thought realistic or based on assumptions?

7. **Consider Environmental Factors**
   External influences can subtly trigger anxiety. Take note of:
   - Who you are with when you feel anxious.
   - The time of day or setting.
   - Whether external stressors, like noise or lighting, contribute to your feelings.

Using Triggers to Your Advantage

Once you've identified your triggers, you can begin to address them:

- **Plan Ahead**: If you know certain situations will provoke anxiety, prepare coping strategies, like deep breathing or grounding exercises, to use in the moment.
- **Set Boundaries**: Limit exposure to avoidable triggers, such as overly critical individuals or stressful environments.
- **Gradual Exposure**: For unavoidable triggers, like social anxiety, gradual exposure can help you build tolerance over time.
- **Challenge Negative Thoughts**: Replace irrational fears with more realistic, balanced perspectives through practices like cognitive-behavioral therapy (CBT).

Identifying your triggers takes time and self-reflection, but the rewards are significant. By shining a light on the sources of your anxiety, you gain the power to disrupt the automatic reactions that fuel it. In the next section, we'll explore how to develop healthy coping mechanisms to respond effectively to your anxiety when it arises.

The Importance of Self-Awareness

Self-awareness is the foundation for understanding and managing anxiety. It is the ability to recognize and understand your thoughts, emotions, behaviors, and how they interact. Developing self-awareness allows you to pinpoint the root of your anxiety, observe how it affects your daily life, and ultimately gain control over your responses. Without self-awareness, anxiety can feel like an uncontrollable force. With it, you can identify patterns, uncover triggers, and implement strategies to reduce its impact.

What is Self-Awareness?

At its core, self-awareness involves two key components:

1. **Internal Self-Awareness**: Understanding your inner world, including your emotions, motivations, and thought patterns.
2. **External Self-Awareness**: Recognizing how your behavior impacts others and how they perceive you.

When it comes to anxiety, both aspects are critical. Internal self-awareness helps you identify when and why you feel anxious, while external self-awareness helps you understand how your reactions may influence your relationships or work environment.

Why Self-Awareness Matters for Anxiety

1. **Recognizing Early Warning Signs**
   Self-awareness allows you to detect anxiety before it spirals out of control. By noticing early warning signs—such as tension in your body, racing thoughts, or irritability—you can intervene with coping strategies before the anxiety becomes overwhelming.
2. **Understanding Your Triggers**
   Becoming self-aware helps you see patterns in your anxiety. By identifying situations, thoughts, or experiences that consistently provoke anxious feelings, you can take proactive steps to address them or minimize their impact.
3. **Breaking Negative Cycles**
   Anxiety often leads to unhelpful thought patterns or behaviors, such as catastrophizing or avoidance. Self-awareness enables you to recognize these tendencies and replace them with healthier habits, such as challenging negative thoughts or practicing gradual exposure to fears.
4. **Improving Emotional Regulation**
   Anxiety can cause emotional outbursts, such as irritability or tearfulness. Self-awareness helps you pause, observe your emotional state, and respond thoughtfully rather than reacting impulsively.
5. **Strengthening Relationships**
   Anxiety doesn't just affect you—it also impacts the people around you. Self-awareness helps you

communicate your needs, set boundaries, and foster understanding in your relationships.

How to Cultivate Self-Awareness

1. **Practice Mindfulness**
   Mindfulness involves paying attention to the present moment without judgment. It helps you notice your thoughts, emotions, and physical sensations as they arise. Techniques include:
   - **Breathing Exercises**: Focus on the rhythm of your breath to calm your mind and observe your body.
   - **Body Scans**: Gradually bring awareness to each part of your body, noticing tension or discomfort.
   - **Mindful Journaling**: Write down your thoughts and feelings to better understand patterns in your anxiety.
2. **Reflect Regularly**
   Spend time reflecting on your day and how anxiety may have influenced your experiences. Ask yourself:
   - When did I feel anxious today?
   - What was happening in that moment?
   - How did I respond, and how might I handle it differently next time?
3. **Seek Feedback**
   Sometimes others notice patterns in our behavior that we miss. Trusted friends, family members, or therapists can

provide valuable insights into how anxiety affects you and your interactions with others.
4. **Identify Your Thought Patterns**
Anxiety often stems from distorted thought patterns, such as all-or-nothing thinking or jumping to conclusions. Keep a log of your anxious thoughts and challenge their validity by asking:
    - Is this thought based on facts or assumptions?
    - What evidence supports or contradicts it?
    - What's a more balanced way to view this situation?
5. **Set Aside Judgment**
Self-awareness is not about criticizing yourself but understanding yourself with curiosity and compassion. When you notice anxious thoughts or behaviors, avoid self-blame and instead focus on what you can learn from the experience.

The Long-Term Benefits of Self-Awareness

Developing self-awareness is an ongoing process, but its rewards are profound:

- **Increased Confidence**: Understanding yourself reduces uncertainty and builds self-trust.
- **Improved Coping Skills**: Recognizing your needs and triggers enables you to use targeted strategies to manage anxiety.

- **Deeper Relationships**: Self-awareness fosters better communication, empathy, and emotional connection with others.
- **Greater Resilience**: By becoming more attuned to your emotions, you can face challenges with clarity and composure.

Self-awareness is the compass that guides you through the complexities of anxiety. In the next section, we'll explore how self-awareness can be used to develop personalized coping strategies that empower you to take control of your mental well-being.

Keeping a Journal: Tracking Your Thoughts and Feelings

A journal is one of the most powerful tools for managing anxiety and gaining insight into your inner world. Writing down your thoughts and emotions allows you to externalize your feelings, identify patterns, and track your progress over time. Journaling is a simple but effective way to develop self-awareness and take control of your mental health.

Why Journaling Helps

1. **Clarifies Thoughts and Emotions**
   When anxiety clouds your mind, it can be difficult to untangle your thoughts. Journaling provides a structured

space to sort through your feelings, offering clarity and a sense of relief.

2. **Identifies Patterns and Triggers**
   By documenting your experiences regularly, you can uncover recurring themes that contribute to your anxiety. This includes specific situations, people, or even internal thoughts that act as triggers.

3. **Reduces Emotional Intensity**
   Putting your feelings into words helps to diffuse their intensity. Studies show that labeling emotions can decrease the activity in the brain's amygdala, which is responsible for fear and emotional reactivity.

4. **Tracks Progress**
   A journal allows you to look back and see how far you've come. Over time, you may notice that situations that once caused anxiety no longer have the same power over you.

How to Start Journaling for Anxiety

1. **Choose a Medium**
   Decide whether you prefer a physical notebook, a digital app, or even voice recordings. Choose a format that feels natural and accessible to you.

2. **Set Aside Time**
   Establish a regular time to journal, whether it's in the morning to set intentions or at night to reflect on the day. Even just 5–10 minutes can make a difference.

3. **Create a Safe Space**
   Journaling is a private activity, so ensure you're in a comfortable and confidential environment where you can write freely.

What to Write About

1. **Daily Reflections**
   Write about your day:
   - What went well?
   - What didn't go as planned?
   - How did you feel during different moments?
2. This practice helps you identify positive moments and areas for improvement.
3. **Anxiety Episodes**
   When you feel anxious, document the experience in detail:
   - What triggered the anxiety?
   - What thoughts went through your mind?
   - How did your body feel (e.g., tense, shaky)?
   - How did you respond, and what helped?
4. Over time, this data can help you see patterns and develop strategies to manage similar situations.
5. **Gratitude Lists**
   Anxiety often narrows focus onto fears and worries. Writing a list of things you're grateful for helps shift your mindset to a more positive and balanced perspective.

6. **Thought Challenging**
   Record an anxious thought and challenge it:
   - Is this thought based on facts or assumptions?
   - What evidence supports or contradicts it?
   - How might a friend or neutral observer view this situation?
7. **Goals and Intentions**
   Set small, manageable goals to help address your anxiety. For example, if you avoid public speaking, your journal can outline steps to gradually face this fear, such as practicing with a trusted friend.

Tips for Effective Journaling

1. **Be Honest**
   Write without censoring yourself. Your journal is a judgment-free zone where you can express your deepest thoughts and feelings.
2. **Write Freely**
   Don't worry about grammar or structure. The goal is to get your thoughts out, not to create a polished piece of writing.
3. **Include Positives**
   While it's important to acknowledge your challenges, also take time to reflect on your strengths, achievements, and moments of joy.
4. **Review Occasionally**
   Periodically read past entries to gain insight into your

progress. This can be motivating and help you recognize how much you've grown.

The Long-Term Benefits of Journaling

Journaling is not just a way to document your experiences—it's a tool for transformation. Over time, it can help you:

- Understand and manage your anxiety triggers.
- Build emotional resilience by identifying and addressing unhelpful thought patterns.
- Foster self-compassion through reflection and self-awareness.
- Develop actionable coping strategies tailored to your unique needs.

By committing to this simple practice, you'll create a roadmap for navigating your anxiety with greater clarity and confidence. In the next section, we'll explore additional strategies for building a personalized anxiety management plan.

Subjective Units of Distress (SUD) Scale

The Subjective Units of Distress (SUD) scale is a simple yet powerful tool for measuring and managing anxiety in real-time. Developed by psychologist Joseph Wolpe, the SUD scale allows you to assign a numerical value to your level of distress, making it easier to track your emotional state and implement coping strategies effectively.

The scale ranges from 0 to 10, with 0 representing complete calm and 10 signifying extreme distress. This tool is particularly useful for recognizing patterns, understanding triggers, and evaluating the effectiveness of interventions.

How the SUD Scale Works

The SUD scale is subjective, meaning it's based entirely on your perception of your emotional state at a given moment. Here's a general breakdown of the scale:

- **0**: Completely calm, no distress at all.
- **1–3**: Mild distress, manageable discomfort, or slight unease.
- **4–6**: Moderate distress, noticeable anxiety but still under control.
- **7–9**: High distress, significant discomfort, or overwhelming anxiety.
- **10**: Extreme distress, panic, or inability to function.

By assigning a number to your distress, you gain a clearer understanding of how intense your emotions are and whether immediate action is needed. Next we will discuss how to use the scale.

1. **Identifying Anxiety Levels**
   Use the scale throughout the day to check in with yourself. Ask, *"What is my current SUD level?"* This practice helps you become more attuned to your emotional state and recognize fluctuations in anxiety.
2. **During Anxiety Episodes**
   When you feel anxious, rate your distress before, during, and after using a coping strategy. This can help you assess the effectiveness of the technique and refine your approach over time.
3. **Tracking Triggers**
   Record your SUD scores alongside triggers in a journal. Over time, patterns will emerge, revealing which situations or thoughts consistently elevate your distress.
4. **Guiding Exposure Therapy**
   For those gradually confronting fears (e.g., through exposure therapy), the SUD scale can measure progress. Starting with lower-stress situations (SUD 3–4) and working up to higher-stress ones (SUD 7–8) allows you to build tolerance at a manageable pace.

How to Incorporate the SUD Scale

1. **Pause and Check In**
   When you notice signs of anxiety, take a moment to pause and ask yourself:
   - What number would I assign to my current level of distress?
   - Why did I choose this number?

- What thoughts, sensations, or external factors are contributing to my score?

2. **Record and Reflect**

   Keeping a log of your SUD scores provides valuable insight into your emotional patterns. For each entry, note:
   - The SUD score.
   - The context (e.g., what was happening or what you were thinking).
   - Any coping strategies you used and how effective they were.

3. **Use Scores to Guide Action**
   - For **low scores (0–3)**: Acknowledge and enjoy your calm state. This is a good time to practice relaxation techniques to reinforce your sense of peace.
   - For **moderate scores (4–6)**: Engage in grounding exercises, such as deep breathing or mindfulness, to prevent anxiety from escalating.
   - For **high scores (7–10)**: Focus on immediate coping strategies, such as removing yourself from the trigger, practicing progressive muscle relaxation, or seeking support from a trusted person.

4. **Reassess After Coping**

   After using a coping strategy, reassess your SUD level. Has the number decreased? If not, consider trying a different technique or taking additional steps to reduce your distress.

Benefits of Using the SUD Scale

1. **Increased Self-Awareness**
   Regularly using the SUD scale helps you become more in tune with your emotional states and identify subtle shifts in anxiety levels.
2. **Improved Coping**
   By rating your distress before and after coping techniques, you can discover which strategies are most effective for you.
3. **Empowerment**
   Assigning a number to your distress can make anxiety feel more manageable. It gives you a concrete way to measure progress and see that distress is not permanent.
4. **Supports Communication**
   The SUD scale can help you communicate your feelings to others. For example, telling a friend or therapist, *"I'm feeling like a 7 right now,"* provides a clear snapshot of your current state.

The SUD scale is a versatile tool that transforms the abstract experience of anxiety into something tangible and measurable. By integrating it into your daily routine, you gain greater control over your emotional well-being and a clearer path to reducing distress. In the next section, we'll explore grounding techniques that pair effectively with the SUD scale to bring your distress levels down in the moment.

Narrative Therapy and Self - Awareness

Narrative therapy is a collaborative, empowering approach that helps individuals reframe their personal stories. At its core, narrative therapy emphasizes the role of storytelling in shaping our identities, beliefs, and experiences. When applied to anxiety, it enables people to gain awareness of how they view themselves in relation to their struggles and to rewrite their narratives in ways that foster resilience, self-compassion, and hope.

This method encourages you to see anxiety not as an intrinsic part of who you are but as an external challenge that you can address and overcome. By becoming aware of the stories you tell yourself and their impact on your emotions, you can reshape your inner dialogue and reclaim control over your life.

The Connection Between Narrative Therapy and Awareness

1. **Understanding Your Story**
   Every individual has a personal narrative—a way of making sense of the events in their life. When anxiety dominates, these stories often become negative, reinforcing feelings of helplessness, fear, or inadequacy. Narrative therapy fosters awareness by helping you examine:

- How do you describe your anxiety?
- What words or metaphors do you use to talk about your experiences?
- Are these stories empowering or limiting?

2. **Separating Yourself from Anxiety**
   A key principle of narrative therapy is *externalization*—viewing anxiety as something separate from yourself, rather than a defining characteristic. For example, instead of saying, *"I'm an anxious person,"* you might say, *"Anxiety sometimes interferes with my life."* This shift in perspective creates space for self-compassion and problem-solving.

3. **Highlighting Strengths and Achievements**
   Narrative therapy also involves identifying the *exceptions*—times when anxiety didn't control your actions or when you successfully managed it. These moments become the building blocks for a new, more empowering narrative about your ability to handle challenges.

Steps to Use Narrative Therapy for Anxiety

1. **Define Your Current Story**
   Start by reflecting on how you currently view anxiety:
   - How would you describe your relationship with anxiety?

- What role does it play in your life (e.g., a barrier, a warning signal, an ever-present force)?
- How has it shaped your decisions, relationships, and identity?

2. Writing this story in a journal can provide valuable insights.

3. **Externalize the Problem**

   Give anxiety its own identity. Some people find it helpful to personify their anxiety as a character or entity. For instance:
   - What would anxiety look like if it were a person or creature?
   - What does it say to you, and how does it behave?
   - How do you respond when it shows up?

4. Externalizing anxiety helps you see it as a challenge to overcome rather than a flaw within yourself.

5. **Identify Exceptions and Strengths**

   Think about times when anxiety didn't hold you back:
   - When have you felt confident or calm despite anxiety's presence?
   - What strategies or resources helped you in those moments?
   - What does this say about your ability to face challenges?

6. Highlighting these exceptions reminds you that anxiety isn't all-powerful and that you have the tools to manage it.

7. **Rewrite Your Narrative**
   Using the insights gained, begin crafting a new, empowering story about your relationship with anxiety. For example:
   - Instead of, *"I'm someone who can't handle stress,"* try, *"I've faced stressful situations before and found ways to cope. Each challenge teaches me something new."*
   - Replace, *"Anxiety ruins everything,"* with, *"Anxiety is something I'm learning to navigate, and I'm getting stronger with each step."*
8. **Share Your Story**
   Sharing your rewritten narrative with a trusted friend, therapist, or even in a journal solidifies your new perspective. Speaking it aloud helps reinforce the empowering aspects of your story.

Benefits of Narrative Therapy for Anxiety

1. **Increased Self-Awareness**
   Examining your personal story helps you recognize the role of anxiety in your life and how your thoughts and beliefs contribute to it.
2. **Empowerment and Agency**
   By reframing your narrative, you shift from feeling like a passive victim of anxiety to an active participant in your own growth and healing.

3. **Strengthened Resilience**
   Focusing on your strengths and past successes builds confidence in your ability to face future challenges.
4. **Reduced Stigma and Self-Blame**
   Externalizing anxiety as something separate from yourself reduces feelings of shame or inadequacy, fostering greater self-compassion.

Practical Tips for Incorporating Narrative Therapy

- **Journal Your Progress**: Keep track of your evolving narrative and the steps you're taking to manage anxiety.
- **Revisit and Revise**: As you grow, your narrative may change. Allow yourself to update your story to reflect your progress and newfound understanding.
- **Pair with Other Techniques**: Narrative therapy works well alongside practices like mindfulness, grounding exercises, and cognitive-behavioral therapy (CBT) to address anxiety from multiple angles.

By becoming the author of your own story, you can transform the way you relate to anxiety. Narrative therapy offers a pathway to greater awareness, resilience, and hope, reminding you that you are more than your struggles and that you have the power to shape your future.

Chapter 4: Coping Strategies and Techniques

Anxiety is a natural response to stress, but when it becomes overwhelming, it can interfere with daily life and well-being. Coping strategies and techniques are practical tools that empower you to manage anxiety, reduce its intensity, and regain control. While no single approach works for everyone, experimenting with a variety of strategies can help you find the methods that suit your needs and lifestyle.

This chapter explores evidence-based techniques to help you face anxiety with confidence and resilience. From immediate tools for calming your mind to long-term strategies for building emotional strength, the following approaches are designed to support your mental health journey.

Immediate Coping Techniques

When anxiety strikes, these quick interventions can help you ground yourself and reduce distress in the moment.

1. **Deep Breathing**
    - **Why It Works**: Deep breathing activates the parasympathetic nervous system, calming your body and mind.
    - **How to Practice**:
        - Inhale deeply through your nose for a count of four.
        - Hold your breath for a count of seven.

- Exhale slowly through your mouth, with tongue positioned on the roof of your mouth, touching the back of your upper front teeth for a count of eight.
- Repeat the cycle four times, focusing on the rhythm of your breath.

2. **Grounding Exercises**
   - **Why It Works**: Grounding redirects your focus from anxious thoughts to the present moment.
   - **How to Practice**:
     - Use the **5-4-3-2-1 Technique**: Identify 5 things you see, 4 things you feel, 3 things you hear, 2 things you smell, and 1 thing you taste.
     - Engage your senses with a calming object, like a textured stone or a scented lotion.

3. **Progressive Muscle Relaxation (PMR)**
   - **Why It Works**: PMR relieves physical tension that often accompanies anxiety.
   - **How to Practice**:
     - Tense each muscle group in your body for 5–10 seconds, then release.
     - Start with your toes and gradually work up to your head.

4. **Visualization**
   - **Why It Works**: Imagining a peaceful scene can shift your mental state.
   - **How to Practice**:

- Close your eyes and picture a serene location, like a beach or forest.
- Engage your senses by imagining the sounds, smells, and textures of the environment.

Long-Term Coping Strategies

Building resilience to anxiety requires consistent effort and self-care. These techniques address the root causes of anxiety and foster emotional balance over time.

1. **Exercise and Physical Activity**
   - **Why It Works**: Exercise reduces stress hormones, releases endorphins, and improves overall mood.
   - **How to Practice**:
     - Aim for at least 30 minutes of moderate exercise most days of the week. Activities like walking, yoga, and swimming can be particularly calming.
2. **Mindfulness and Meditation**
   - **Why It Works**: Mindfulness helps you observe anxious thoughts without judgment, reducing their hold on you.
   - **How to Practice**:
     - Try a guided meditation app or practice mindfulness by focusing on your breath or bodily sensations for 5–10 minutes a day.

Sleep Hygiene
- **Why It Works**: Quality sleep restores your body and mind, making you more resilient to stress.
- **How to Practice**:
  - Maintain a consistent sleep schedule.
  - Avoid screens and stimulating activities an hour before bed.
  - Create a calming bedtime routine, such as reading or practicing relaxation exercises.

3. Healthy Diet
- **Why It Works**: A balanced diet supports brain health and regulates mood.
- **How to Practice**:
  - Eat regular meals with plenty of fruits, vegetables, whole grains, and lean proteins.
  - Limit caffeine, sugar, and processed foods, which can exacerbate anxiety.

4. Cognitive-Behavioral Strategies
- **Why It Works**: Challenging unhelpful thought patterns reduces the mental spiral that fuels anxiety.
- **How to Practice**:
  - Identify negative thoughts, question their validity, and replace them with balanced alternatives.

Since anxiety can manifest in different ways, having a diverse set of coping strategies is essential. Here are tips for building your personalized toolkit:

1. **Experiment with Techniques**
    - Try various strategies to see what resonates with you. For example, if deep breathing feels too abstract, grounding exercises might be more effective.
2. **Combine Methods**
    - Pair immediate techniques (e.g., breathing exercises) with long-term practices (e.g., mindfulness or exercise) for comprehensive support.
3. **Prepare for Triggers**
    - Identify situations that typically provoke anxiety and plan coping strategies in advance.
4. **Practice Regularly**
    - Like any skill, coping strategies become more effective with consistent practice, even when you're not feeling anxious.
5. **Seek Support**
    - Don't hesitate to involve a therapist, counselor, or support group to enhance your toolkit and gain professional guidance.

The Role of Self-Compassion

Coping with anxiety is a journey, not a destination. Along the way, you may experience setbacks, but it's crucial to approach yourself with kindness and patience. Remember that anxiety is not a reflection of your worth—it's a natural response that can be managed with the right tools and support.

In the next section, we'll delve into specific lifestyle adjustments that complement these coping strategies and create a foundation for long-term mental well-being.

Breathing Exercises for Immediate Relief

When anxiety strikes, it often manifests physically through rapid, shallow breathing, a racing heart, or a tight chest. These symptoms are the result of your body activating its *fight-or-flight* response, preparing you to face a perceived threat. However, in most situations, the threat isn't physical—it's emotional or mental. Breathing exercises are a simple, effective way to counteract this response by calming your nervous system and signaling to your brain that you are safe.

By focusing on your breath, you can shift your body out of an anxious state and into a more relaxed one. Here are some of the most effective breathing exercises for immediate anxiety relief.

1. Box Breathing

Box breathing, also known as square breathing, is a structured breathing technique that helps regulate your breath and calm your mind.

- **How to Practice**:
    1. Inhale deeply through your nose for a count of 4.
    2. Hold your breath for a count of 4.
    3. Exhale slowly through your mouth for a count of 4.
    4. Hold your breath again for a count of 4.
    5. Repeat this cycle 4–5 times, focusing on the even rhythm of your breath.
- **Why It Works**: The steady rhythm of box breathing soothes the nervous system and provides a sense of control, which can be especially comforting during moments of anxiety.

2. 4-7-8 Breathing

The 4-7-8 method is a calming technique often used to reduce stress and promote relaxation.

- **How to Practice**:
    1. Inhale through your nose for a count of 4.
    2. Hold your breath for a count of 7.
    3. Exhale completely through your mouth for a count of 8, making a whooshing sound.
    4. Repeat the cycle for 4–5 breaths.

- **Why It Works**: By extending the exhale longer than the inhale, this technique encourages your body to enter a relaxed state, counteracting anxiety-induced hyperventilation.

3. Diaphragmatic Breathing

Also known as belly breathing, this technique engages the diaphragm, a large muscle at the base of your lungs, to promote deep and efficient breathing.

- **How to Practice**:
    1. Sit or lie down in a comfortable position. Place one hand on your chest and the other on your abdomen.
    2. Inhale deeply through your nose, allowing your abdomen to rise as you fill your lungs with air. Your chest should remain still.
    3. Exhale slowly through your mouth, letting your abdomen fall.
    4. Continue for 5–10 minutes, focusing on the rise and fall of your abdomen.
- **Why It Works**: Diaphragmatic breathing slows your heart rate and reduces physical tension, creating a sense of calm.

This breathing exercise helps balance the mind and body by alternating airflow through each nostril.

- **How to Practice**:
    1. Sit comfortably with your back straight.
    2. Using your thumb, close your right nostril and inhale deeply through your left nostril.
    3. Close your left nostril with your ring finger, release your thumb, and exhale through your right nostril.
    4. Inhale through your right nostril, then close it and exhale through your left nostril.
    5. Repeat this cycle for 1–3 minutes.
- **Why It Works**: This practice calms the mind, reduces anxiety, and enhances focus by encouraging balanced breathing.

4. Resonance Breathing (Coherent Breathing)

Resonance breathing involves maintaining a slow, steady breathing rate to achieve a state of relaxation and balance.

- **How to Practice**:
    1. Inhale slowly through your nose for a count of 5.
    2. Exhale gently through your mouth for a count of 5.
    3. Continue this rhythm for 5–10 minutes, keeping your breaths smooth and even.
- **Why It Works**: Resonance breathing lowers blood pressure and reduces the activity of the stress response system, helping you feel calm and centered.

Tips for Success

- **Find a Quiet Space**: While you can practice breathing exercises anywhere, a quiet and comfortable environment can enhance their effectiveness.
- **Focus on Your Breath**: Pay attention to the sensation of air entering and leaving your body. If your mind wanders, gently bring your focus back to your breathing.
- **Practice Regularly**: Incorporating these exercises into your daily routine can help you respond to anxiety more effectively when it arises.
- **Pair with Visualization**: Combine breathing exercises with calming imagery, such as picturing waves gently lapping on a shore, to deepen relaxation.

When to Use Breathing Exercises

Breathing exercises are versatile and can be used in a variety of situations:

- **During an Anxiety Episode**: To regain control and reduce symptoms.
- **Before a Stressful Event**: Such as a presentation, interview, or test, to calm preemptive nerves.
- **As a Daily Practice**: To build resilience and maintain a sense of balance.

Breathing is a tool you always have with you, making it one of the most accessible and reliable strategies for managing anxiety. In the next section, we'll explore grounding techniques that complement breathing exercises to help you feel more present and in control during anxious moments.

Mindfulness and Meditation Practices

Mindfulness and meditation are transformative practices that can help manage anxiety by bringing attention to the present moment and cultivating a sense of calm and awareness. These techniques empower you to observe your thoughts and feelings without judgment, reducing the hold of anxious patterns and promoting inner peace.

Anxiety often thrives in the "what-ifs" of the future or the regrets of the past. Mindfulness and meditation redirect focus to the present, breaking the cycle of rumination and worry. This section delves into practical methods to incorporate mindfulness and meditation into your daily routine.

The Science Behind Mindfulness and Meditation

Research has shown that mindfulness and meditation can significantly reduce symptoms of anxiety by:

- **Lowering Stress Hormones**: Practices like meditation decrease cortisol levels, the hormone associated with stress.

- **Rewiring the Brain**: Regular meditation enhances neuroplasticity, improving the brain's ability to adapt and regulate emotions.
- **Activating the Relaxation Response**: These practices calm the fight-or-flight system, promoting a state of relaxation.

Key Mindfulness Practices

1. **Mindful Breathing**
    - **What It Is**: Paying attention to the natural rhythm of your breath.
    - **How to Practice**:
        1. Sit comfortably in a quiet space.
        2. Close your eyes or soften your gaze.
        3. Focus on the sensation of air entering and leaving your nostrils or the rise and fall of your chest.
        4. If your mind wanders, gently guide it back to your breath.
    - **Why It Works**: Anchoring attention to the breath prevents your mind from spiraling into anxious thoughts.
2. **Body Scan**
    - **What It Is**: A practice of observing physical sensations throughout your body.
    - **How to Practice**:
        1. Lie down or sit in a comfortable position.

2. Close your eyes and take a few deep breaths.
3. Slowly move your attention through each part of your body, starting from your toes and working up to your head.
4. Notice any tension or discomfort, and consciously release it.
- **Why It Works**: A body scan connects you to physical sensations, grounding you in the present and promoting relaxation.

3. **Five Senses Exercise**
   - **What It Is**: A grounding technique using sensory awareness.
   - **How to Practice**: Identify:
     1. 5 things you can see,
     2. 4 things you can feel,
     3. 3 things you can hear,
     4. 2 things you can smell, and
     5. 1 thing you can taste.
   - **Why It Works**: Engaging the senses redirects focus away from anxious thoughts and into the here and now.

4. **Mindful Walking**
   - **What It Is**: Bringing awareness to the act of walking.
   - **How to Practice**:
     1. Walk slowly in a quiet space.
     2. Focus on the sensation of your feet touching the ground, the rhythm of your steps, and your surroundings.

3. Notice any thoughts or feelings that arise, letting them pass without judgment.
- **Why It Works**: Movement paired with mindfulness can soothe the mind and release physical tension.

Meditation Techniques for Anxiety

1. **Loving-Kindness Meditation (Metta)**
   - **What It Is**: A practice of cultivating compassion for yourself and others.
   - **How to Practice**:
     1. Sit comfortably and close your eyes.
     2. Silently repeat phrases such as, *"May I be happy. May I be healthy. May I be safe."*
     3. Extend these wishes to loved ones, acquaintances, and even those you struggle with.
   - **Why It Works**: Fostering positive emotions helps counteract negative thought patterns associated with anxiety.
2. **Guided Visualization**
   - **What It Is**: Using imagery to evoke a sense of calm.
   - **How to Practice**:
     1. Listen to a guided meditation or visualize a peaceful scene, such as a beach or forest.
     2. Engage your senses by imagining the sounds, smells, and textures of the environment.

- **Why It Works**: Visualization engages the imagination, offering a mental escape from anxiety-provoking thoughts.

3. **Mantra Meditation**
    - **What It Is**: Repeating a calming word or phrase.
    - **How to Practice**:
        1. Choose a word or phrase like *"peace," "calm,"* or *"I am safe."*
        2. Silently repeat the mantra during meditation, synchronizing it with your breath.
    - **Why It Works**: The repetition of a mantra focuses your mind and creates a sense of stability.

4. **Mindfulness of Thoughts**
    - **What It Is**: Observing thoughts without becoming attached to them.
    - **How to Practice**:
        1. Sit quietly and notice any thoughts that arise.
        2. Label them as *"thought," "feeling,"* or *"sensation,"* and let them pass like clouds in the sky.
    - **Why It Works**: Recognizing thoughts as transient reduces their power over you.

Tips for Building a Mindfulness and Meditation Practice

1. **Start Small**
    - Begin with just 5 minutes a day and gradually increase the duration as you feel comfortable.

2. **Create a Routine**
   - Meditate at the same time each day, such as in the morning or before bed, to establish a habit.
3. **Be Patient**
   - Mindfulness and meditation are skills that develop with practice. It's okay if your mind wanders—what matters is bringing it back.
4. **Use Resources**
   - Explore apps like Headspace, Calm, or Insight Timer for guided meditations.
5. **Combine with Other Practices**
   - Pair mindfulness with breathing exercises, yoga, or journaling to enhance its effectiveness.

By incorporating mindfulness and meditation into your life, you can build a stronger foundation for managing anxiety. These practices teach you to respond to anxious thoughts with clarity and composure, empowering you to face challenges with greater ease. In the next section, we'll explore the importance of cultivating a support system as part of your anxiety management plan.

Grounding Techniques for Panic Attacks

Panic attacks can feel overwhelming, both physically and emotionally. Symptoms like a racing heart, shortness of breath, dizziness, and a sense of impending doom can make you feel out of control. Grounding techniques are powerful tools for managing these episodes, as they help anchor you to the present moment and redirect your focus away from the intense sensations of panic.

Grounding techniques work by engaging your senses and interrupting the mental loop of fear and distress. Here, we'll explore practical strategies to help you regain control during a panic attack.

What Are Grounding Techniques?

Grounding techniques are exercises designed to help you reconnect with your body, surroundings, and present reality. They're particularly effective during panic attacks because they create a mental and physical "pause," helping to calm your nervous system.

Grounding Techniques to Try

1. **The 5-4-3-2-1 Method**
    - **What It Is**: A sensory awareness exercise to focus your mind on your environment.
    - **How to Practice**:
        - Name 5 things you can see around you.
        - Name 4 things you can physically feel (e.g., your feet on the ground, the texture of your clothing).
        - Name 3 things you can hear.

- Name 2 things you can smell (or imagine smells you enjoy).
- Name 1 thing you can taste (or imagine a comforting taste).
  - **Why It Works**: Engaging your senses pulls your attention away from your internal panic and reconnects you with your surroundings.

2. **Cold Sensation Technique**
   - **What It Is**: Using a cold object or sensation to ground yourself.
   - **How to Practice**:
     - Hold an ice cube in your hand or run cold water over your wrists.
     - Focus on the sensation of coldness and how it feels against your skin.
   - **Why It Works**: The intense physical sensation interrupts racing thoughts and shifts your focus.

3. **Grounding with Touch**
   - **What It Is**: Using physical objects to bring yourself back to the present.
   - **How to Practice**:
     - Grab a textured object (e.g., a stress ball, a smooth stone, or fabric).
     - Notice the texture, temperature, and weight of the object in your hands.
   - **Why It Works**: Focusing on tactile sensations distracts your mind from panic symptoms.

4. **Feet-on-the-Ground Technique**

- **What It Is**: Using the sensation of your feet against the floor to feel rooted.
- **How to Practice**:
  - Sit or stand comfortably and place your feet flat on the ground.
  - Press your feet into the floor, noticing the firmness and support beneath you.
  - Wiggle your toes or shift your weight slightly to enhance the connection.
- **Why It Works**: Feeling physically grounded can counteract the sense of floating or losing control common during panic attacks.

5. **Breathing with Counting**
   - **What It Is**: Combining deep breathing with mental focus.
   - **How to Practice**:
     - Inhale deeply through your nose for a count of 4.
     - Hold your breath for a count of 4.
     - Exhale slowly through your mouth for a count of 6.
     - Repeat for several cycles, focusing on the count and the rhythm of your breath.
   - **Why It Works**: Counting adds a cognitive task, distracting your mind from the panic while calming your body.

6. **Describing Your Environment**

- **What It Is**: Verbally or mentally describing your surroundings in detail.
- **How to Practice**:
  - Look around and describe what you see, such as the color of the walls, the shapes of objects, or the lighting in the room.
  - Include as much detail as possible, focusing on neutral or calming elements.
- **Why It Works**: Shifting your focus to neutral observations helps create a mental distance from panic.

7. **Mantras and Affirmations**
   - **What It Is**: Using calming phrases to reassure yourself.
   - **How to Practice**:
     - Repeat phrases like, *"This is temporary. I am safe. I will get through this."*
     - Say it out loud or silently, aligning the words with your breathing.
   - **Why It Works**: Reassuring words can reduce fear and reinforce a sense of control.

8. **Physical Movement**
   - **What It Is**: Engaging your body in simple, repetitive motion.
   - **How to Practice**:
     - Walk slowly and deliberately, paying attention to each step.

- ■ Stretch your arms, legs, or neck, focusing on how your muscles feel as they move.
  - ○ **Why It Works**: Movement provides a physical outlet for tension and redirects nervous energy.

Tips for Using Grounding Techniques

- **Practice Regularly**: Familiarize yourself with these techniques during calm moments so they're easier to use during a panic attack.
- **Create a Grounding Toolkit**: Keep a small box with grounding items like a stress ball, essential oils, or a list of affirmations.
- **Be Patient**: It might take a few minutes for the techniques to take effect. Stick with them and trust the process.
- **Combine Methods**: You can mix techniques, such as combining breathing exercises with sensory grounding, for added effectiveness.

When to Use Grounding Techniques

- **During a Panic Attack**: To regain a sense of control and reduce distress.
- **In Triggering Situations**: If you anticipate an anxiety-provoking event, grounding can help you stay calm.

- **As Part of Daily Practice**: Incorporating grounding into your routine can make it easier to access in moments of high anxiety.

Grounding techniques are simple yet powerful tools for managing panic attacks. By anchoring yourself to the present, you can navigate these intense moments with greater confidence and ease. In the next section, we'll explore the role of lifestyle changes in supporting long-term anxiety management.

Progressive Muscle Relaxation (PMR)

Progressive Muscle Relaxation (PMR) is a simple yet highly effective technique designed to reduce anxiety and stress by focusing on tensing and relaxing different muscle groups in the body. It helps you become more aware of physical tension, which is often a result of anxiety, and teaches you how to release it. By actively relaxing muscles one at a time, PMR can have a calming effect on the nervous system, making it an excellent tool for managing panic attacks, stress, and general anxiety.

What is Progressive Muscle Relaxation?

PMR was developed by Dr. Edmund Jacobson in the early 1920s as a way to reduce stress and improve overall health. The core concept involves systematically tensing and then relaxing specific muscle groups in the body, starting from the toes and working up to the head. This process promotes the awareness of physical tension and teaches the body how to release it.

By practicing PMR, you learn how to recognize and respond to tension in the body, which is a key aspect of managing anxiety. Anxiety often manifests physically, such as muscle tightness, shallow breathing, or a racing heart. PMR counteracts this by intentionally relaxing each muscle group, promoting overall relaxation and well-being.

How to Practice Progressive Muscle Relaxation

1. **Find a Comfortable Position**
   - Sit or lie down in a quiet place where you can relax without distractions. Close your eyes if that helps you focus.
2. **Focus on Your Breath**
   - Before starting, take a few deep breaths to center yourself. Inhale deeply through your nose, allowing your lungs to fill, and then exhale slowly through your mouth. Continue breathing slowly and deeply throughout the practice.
3. **Tense and Relax Each Muscle Group**
   The key to PMR is the contrast between tension and relaxation. For each muscle group, you'll tense the

muscles for 5–10 seconds, then relax them for 20–30 seconds, noticing the difference. Here's how to proceed:
- **Feet and Toes**:
  - Curl your toes tightly and tense the muscles in your feet. Hold for 5–10 seconds.
  - Relax your feet and focus on the release of tension. Feel your feet sinking into the ground or the surface beneath you.
- **Calves**:
  - Flex your feet by pointing your toes upward, tightening the muscles in your calves. Hold for 5–10 seconds.
  - Release the tension and focus on the feeling of relaxation in your calves.
- **Thighs**:
  - Tighten your thigh muscles by pressing your knees together or squeezing your thighs. Hold for 5–10 seconds.
  - Release and feel the relaxation flow through your thighs.
- **Abdomen**:
  - Tighten your abdominal muscles by drawing your belly button in toward your spine. Hold for 5–10 seconds.
  - Relax and let go of the tension.
- **Hands and Arms**:
  - Make fists with both hands and tighten your forearms. Hold for 5–10 seconds.

- Release and notice the relaxation spreading through your hands and arms.
  - **Shoulders**:
    - Lift your shoulders toward your ears, squeezing them tightly. Hold for 5–10 seconds.
    - Relax your shoulders and allow them to drop away from your ears.
  - **Face**:
    - Scrunch your face as tightly as you can by closing your eyes, tightening your forehead, and pursing your lips. Hold for 5–10 seconds.
    - Relax your face and feel the tension melt away.

4. **Move Upward**
   - Work your way up the body, starting from the feet and moving toward the head. The last muscle group should be the face and neck. This progressive approach helps promote a sense of overall relaxation.
5. **Finish with Deep Breathing**
   - Once you've relaxed all the muscle groups, take a few more deep breaths. Allow your body to fully relax, and focus on how your body feels without the tension. Let your muscles feel heavy and completely at ease.

Why Progressive Muscle Relaxation Works for Anxiety

PMR has several psychological and physiological benefits that help alleviate anxiety:

1. **Reduces Physical Tension**: Anxiety often manifests in physical symptoms like tight muscles, shallow breathing, or clenched jaws. PMR teaches you to consciously release tension, helping to break the cycle of physical discomfort.
2. **Activates the Relaxation Response**: The process of tensing and relaxing muscles activates the parasympathetic nervous system, the body's "rest and digest" mode, which counteracts the stress response (fight or flight).
3. **Enhances Mind-Body Connection**: PMR increases body awareness, helping you become more attuned to the physical sensations of anxiety and the signs that your body is in a tense state.
4. **Promotes Calm**: The contrast between tension and relaxation helps create a calming effect on both the mind and body. By practicing PMR regularly, you can use it as a powerful tool during times of stress or anxiety.

Tips for Success

1. **Practice Regularly**: The more you practice PMR, the easier it becomes to notice and manage tension in your

body. Make it part of your daily routine, even if you don't feel anxious.
2. **Be Gentle with Yourself**: If you experience any discomfort while tensing a muscle group, ease up on the tension. The goal is to find a level of tension that is strong but not painful.
3. **Use PMR in Combination**: Pair PMR with other relaxation techniques like deep breathing or guided meditation for a deeper sense of calm.
4. **Practice in a Quiet Environment**: To enhance relaxation, practice PMR in a space free from distractions. Consider dimming the lights or listening to calming music to promote a soothing atmosphere.

When to Use Progressive Muscle Relaxation

- **During a Panic Attack**: If you're experiencing a panic attack, PMR can help you regain a sense of control by releasing physical tension and promoting relaxation.
- **Before Stressful Events**: Use PMR before challenging situations such as public speaking, meetings, or exams to calm your nerves.
- **As Part of a Self-Care Routine**: Incorporate PMR into your daily self-care routine, especially if you have chronic anxiety or stress. Regular practice can help prevent the build-up of tension.

Progressive Muscle Relaxation is a powerful technique.

Chapter 5:Cognitive Behavioral Therapy (CBT)

Cognitive Behavioral Therapy (CBT) is a highly versatile and evidence-based psychological treatment that has been shown to help individuals address a wide range of mental health issues. In this expanded section, we will dive deeper into the fundamental principles of CBT, explore how it works in greater detail, and examine its various applications, strategies, and techniques. We will also look into how CBT can be applied to both individual and group therapy settings and how it can be integrated into other forms of treatment.

Aaron T. Beck is often credited with formally founding Cognitive Therapy (CT) in the 1960s. Beck's approach was grounded in the idea that distorted or negative thinking patterns contribute to emotional problems, particularly depression and anxiety. Beck's clinical work led him to recognize common cognitive distortions—such as catastrophizing and overgeneralizing—that exacerbate emotional distress. He developed tools like the Beck Depression Inventory to assess the severity of depressive symptoms and laid the groundwork for what would later become CBT.

Core Concepts of CBT

The foundational idea behind Cognitive Behavioral Therapy is the belief that our thoughts, feelings, and behaviors are all interconnected, and that by changing one of these components, we can influence the others in a positive direction. This is often referred to as the cognitive triangle.

1. Thoughts: Our cognitive patterns, including how we perceive situations, how we interpret events, and the automatic thoughts that arise in our minds, can significantly influence how we feel and act. These thoughts can be distorted, biased, or unrealistic, leading to negative emotions and maladaptive behaviors.
2. Emotions: Our emotional responses are deeply tied to our thoughts. For instance, if we have negative thoughts, we are likely to experience negative emotions, such as sadness, anger, or anxiety. Conversely, positive thoughts often result in more positive emotional responses.
3. Behaviors: The way we behave is often influenced by our emotions and thoughts. For example, if we are anxious about a social situation (a thought), we may avoid it altogether (a behavior), which in turn reinforces our anxiety.

The goal of CBT is to help individuals break out of negative cycles of thinking, feeling, and behaving by learning new, healthier patterns. CBT is built around the premise that our cognitive distortions (unhelpful or irrational thoughts) can be identified, challenged, and restructured to create more balanced and realistic ways of thinking.

1. Cognitive Restructuring: One of the central techniques in CBT is cognitive restructuring (or cognitive reframing), which involves identifying and challenging negative thoughts. The process includes recognizing distorted thinking, evaluating its accuracy, and replacing it with more realistic and balanced thoughts. Some common examples of distorted thinking patterns include:
     - Overgeneralization: Drawing broad conclusions based on limited evidence.
     - Catastrophizing: Expecting the worst possible outcome without evidence.
     - Personalization: Blaming oneself for events outside one's control.
     - Mind Reading: Assuming you know what others are thinking or feeling, often in a negative light.
2. For example, a person might think, "I always fail at everything I do," which is a form of overgeneralization. In CBT, the therapist would work with the person to examine evidence for and against this thought, helping them to develop a more accurate, balanced perspective, such as, "I've faced challenges before, but I have succeeded in many areas as well."
3. Behavioral Activation: Behavioral activation is a technique used to address the avoidance behaviors often associated with depression and anxiety. When people experience negative emotions, they often withdraw from activities they once enjoyed, leading to a cycle of increasing isolation and decreased mood. In CBT,

individuals are encouraged to engage in pleasant and meaningful activities to disrupt this cycle. This might involve creating a daily or weekly schedule that includes activities they find enjoyable, rewarding, or fulfilling.
4. Exposure Therapy: Exposure therapy is commonly used for individuals with anxiety disorders, particularly phobias, post-traumatic stress disorder (PTSD), and obsessive-compulsive disorder (OCD). The idea behind exposure therapy is to gradually expose individuals to feared situations in a controlled and safe environment, helping them face their fears in a systematic and gradual way. Over time, this helps reduce the anxiety and distress associated with those situations. For example, someone with a fear of flying might start by imagining themselves on a plane, then progress to visiting an airport, and eventually take a short flight.
5. Mindfulness: Although traditionally associated with mindfulness-based therapies, mindfulness practices have also become a key technique in CBT. Mindfulness involves paying attention to the present moment without judgment, helping individuals become more aware of their thoughts, emotions, and physical sensations. In CBT, mindfulness is used to help individuals detach from their negative thoughts, observing them without becoming overwhelmed by them. Mindfulness can be particularly useful for individuals struggling with rumination, anxiety, or intrusive thoughts.

6. Thought Records: Thought records are a valuable tool used in CBT to help individuals track their thoughts and identify patterns. By keeping a daily log of situations that provoke negative emotions, along with the thoughts that accompany them, individuals can identify cognitive distortions and work through them. Thought records often include columns for:
    - The situation: What happened?
    - The thoughts: What thoughts went through your mind?
    - The emotions: What emotions did you feel, and at what intensity?
    - Alternative thoughts: What is a more balanced or realistic thought?
    - New emotions: How do you feel now after challenging the negative thoughts?
7. Problem-Solving: CBT encourages individuals to break down overwhelming problems into manageable steps and to approach them in a solution-focused way. This involves clarifying the problem, brainstorming possible solutions, evaluating pros and cons, and implementing the best course of action. Problem-solving helps people build confidence in their ability to cope with difficulties and reduce feelings of helplessness.

How CBT Works: A Step-by-Step Process

While every individual's experience with CBT may differ, the process typically follows these general steps:

1. Initial Assessment: During the first sessions, the therapist works with the client to understand their challenges, symptoms, and goals. This includes identifying the specific problems they want to address (e.g., anxiety, depression, stress) and creating a plan for treatment.
2. Identifying Negative Thoughts and Behaviors: In subsequent sessions, the therapist helps the individual identify the negative thought patterns and behaviors that contribute to their distress. This might involve exploring past experiences, current situations, and the automatic thoughts that arise in response to these experiences.
3. Challenging and Reframing Thoughts: The therapist and client work together to challenge negative thoughts and replace them with more balanced, positive alternatives. The therapist may use various techniques to help the client evaluate their thoughts, such as asking them to examine evidence for and against their beliefs, considering alternative viewpoints, and exploring the worst-case and best-case scenarios.
4. Changing Behaviors: As part of the therapy, the therapist helps the individual adopt healthier coping strategies, improve problem-solving skills, and increase engagement in rewarding activities. Behavioral activation

is a key technique for addressing the avoidance behaviors often seen in depression and anxiety.
5. Skill Development and Homework: CBT is a highly interactive and practical therapy. Clients are often given homework assignments designed to help them apply what they've learned in sessions to real-life situations. This could include completing thought records, practicing relaxation techniques, engaging in new behaviors, or experimenting with new ways of thinking.
6. Reviewing Progress and Maintenance: Throughout the course of therapy, the therapist and client regularly assess progress. If necessary, adjustments are made to the treatment plan. As therapy progresses, the individual gains greater confidence in managing their thoughts, emotions, and behaviors independently, with the goal of eventually ending therapy and maintaining positive changes on their own.

The Effectiveness of CBT

Cognitive Behavioral Therapy has been shown to be effective in treating a wide range of mental health issues. Its structured, practical approach allows it to address both the cognitive and behavioral aspects of psychological distress, making it a powerful tool for helping individuals with anxiety, depression, OCD, PTSD, and more.

- Evidence-Based: CBT is one of the most well-researched therapeutic approaches. Numerous studies have shown its effectiveness in treating various conditions, including anxiety disorders, depression, eating disorders, and chronic pain.
- Long-Term Benefits: Unlike some therapies that may offer short-term relief, CBT has been shown to provide lasting results. Because it equips individuals with practical tools to manage their thoughts and behaviors, the benefits of CBT often persist long after therapy has ended.
- Adaptability: CBT can be adapted to suit individual needs. It works for both individuals and groups, and can be used alongside other treatments, such as medication or mindfulness-based therapies.

Core Principles of CBT

1. **The Cognitive Triangle**: One of the central tenets of CBT is the **cognitive triangle**, which emphasizes the relationship between **thoughts**, **emotions**, and **behaviors**. The cognitive triangle illustrates how each component influences the others:
    - **Thoughts**: Our perceptions and interpretations of events.
    - **Emotions**: The feelings that arise in response to our thoughts.
    - **Behaviors**: The actions we take in response to our thoughts and emotions.

2. The fundamental idea in CBT is that negative or distorted thoughts can lead to negative emotions and behaviors, which in turn reinforce and perpetuate psychological distress. By identifying and altering these unhelpful thought patterns, individuals can experience significant improvements in how they feel and act.
3. **The Role of Cognitive Distortions**: Cognitive distortions are irrational or biased ways of thinking that contribute to emotional and behavioral problems. Some common examples of cognitive distortions include:
   - **All-or-nothing thinking**: Viewing situations in extreme, black-and-white terms.
   - **Catastrophizing**: Expecting the worst possible outcome.
   - **Mind reading**: Assuming we know what others are thinking or feeling, often in a negative way.
   - **Personalization**: Blaming oneself for things outside one's control.
4. In CBT, individuals learn to recognize these distortions in their thinking, challenge them, and replace them with more balanced and rational thoughts.
5. **The Behavioral Component**: In addition to addressing thought patterns, CBT also involves modifying behaviors that contribute to emotional distress. Often, people engage in avoidance behaviors, such as avoiding social situations because they fear judgment, which can reinforce anxiety and depression. CBT encourages individuals to face their fears gradually through **exposure**

techniques, **behavioral activation**, and **problem-solving strategies**.
- **Behavioral Activation**: This technique is used particularly for depression, where individuals are encouraged to re-engage with enjoyable and meaningful activities to counteract the tendency to withdraw from life and isolate themselves.
- **Exposure Therapy**: For anxiety disorders, exposure therapy involves gradually confronting feared situations or thoughts, helping to desensitize the individual to the anxiety-provoking stimuli and reduce avoidance behavior.

The Benefits of CBT

1. **Effective for a Range of Mental Health Conditions**: CBT has been demonstrated to be effective for a wide variety of mental health issues, making it one of the most widely used and researched therapeutic modalities. These include:
   - **Anxiety disorders** (e.g., generalized anxiety disorder, panic disorder, social anxiety, phobias)
   - **Depression**
   - **Obsessive-compulsive disorder (OCD)**
   - **Post-traumatic stress disorder (PTSD)**
   - **Eating disorders**
   - **Chronic pain** and other physical health issues
   - **Substance use disorders**

- **Anger management**
- **Sleep problems** (e.g., insomnia)
2. CBT's versatility makes it appropriate for a wide range of people and situations. Whether an individual is struggling with a specific phobia or general anxiety, or battling feelings of hopelessness and sadness, CBT provides concrete strategies to tackle these challenges effectively.
3. **Short-Term and Goal-Oriented**: One of the major advantages of CBT is that it is typically a **short-term** therapy compared to other therapeutic approaches. Most CBT treatments last between **8 to 20 sessions**, depending on the severity and complexity of the issues being addressed. The therapy is focused on specific goals, making it results-driven. Individuals work collaboratively with their therapist to set goals, and progress is regularly evaluated. This structured, time-limited approach can be appealing to those who seek clear, tangible outcomes.
4. **Empowering Individuals**: CBT encourages **self-efficacy**, which is the belief in one's ability to influence events in one's life. Through CBT, individuals learn to take an active role in managing their thoughts, emotions, and behaviors. This sense of agency empowers individuals to implement the skills they acquire in therapy in their daily lives, making them less reliant on the therapist once the treatment ends. This self-help aspect makes CBT highly effective for people who want to take charge of their own mental health.

5. **Promotes Long-Term Change**: Unlike some other therapies that focus primarily on understanding the root causes of issues, CBT is practical and forward-focused. By learning how to challenge cognitive distortions, individuals develop lasting coping strategies that can be applied to future challenges. This focus on equipping individuals with lifelong tools to manage stress, anxiety, depression, and other mental health issues has been shown to help prevent relapse and improve overall functioning.
6. **Improves Problem-Solving and Coping Skills**: CBT teaches **problem-solving skills** that help individuals break down complex challenges into manageable steps. These skills are useful in all aspects of life, from managing work-related stress to navigating personal relationships. Additionally, CBT encourages individuals to approach problems in a more **rational** and **structured** manner, reducing emotional reactivity and improving overall decision-making.
7. **Helps Develop Healthier Coping Mechanisms**: In CBT, individuals learn to develop healthier coping strategies to replace maladaptive behaviors such as avoidance, rumination, and self-blame. By using techniques like **relaxation exercises**, **mindfulness**, and **assertiveness training**, individuals can better manage stress and anxiety, improving their emotional resilience in the long run.

8. **Focus on the Present**: CBT places a strong emphasis on the present moment and the here-and-now. While it may involve some exploration of past events to understand how they may be influencing current thinking, the primary focus is on addressing current issues and how to overcome them. This focus on the present helps individuals move away from rumination about past events or worrying about the future, both of which can contribute to anxiety and depression.

How CBT Works: A Practical Example

To better understand how CBT works, let's take a look at a practical example:

Imagine someone named **Jane**, who has been struggling with anxiety about public speaking. Her negative thoughts about public speaking include:

- "I'm going to make a fool of myself."
- "Everyone will judge me."
- "I won't be able to handle it."

These thoughts make Jane feel anxious and scared, leading her to avoid speaking in front of others. This avoidance reinforces her anxiety, making her believe even more strongly that public speaking is something to fear.

In CBT, Jane would work with her therapist to:

1. **Identify and challenge** these negative thoughts. The therapist may help her realize that her fears are exaggerated or unrealistic, and that others are likely not judging her as harshly as she imagines.
2. **Reframe** her thoughts: For example, Jane may begin to challenge her belief by thinking, "It's okay to make mistakes, and most people will be supportive."
3. **Gradual exposure**: Jane might gradually face her fear of public speaking by starting with smaller, less intimidating situations, such as speaking in front of a friend or a small group.
4. **Behavioral activation**: Jane might engage in positive reinforcement strategies, rewarding herself after each public speaking opportunity, reinforcing her progress and building confidence.

By the end of treatment, Jane would not only have developed healthier thinking patterns around public speaking but would also have gained the tools to face similar challenges in the future.

Reframing Negative Thoughts Using CBT

One of the core components of Cognitive Behavioral Therapy (CBT) is **cognitive restructuring**, a process in which individuals learn to identify, challenge, and reframe negative or distorted thoughts. Negative thoughts often lead to feelings of anxiety, depression, and stress, and they can perpetuate unhealthy behaviors. The goal of reframing is to replace these unhelpful thoughts with more balanced, realistic, and helpful alternatives. Here's how the process works:

1. Identifying Negative Thoughts

The first step in reframing negative thoughts is to **become aware of them**. Often, these thoughts occur automatically and without conscious awareness. In CBT, individuals are taught to recognize these thoughts by paying attention to their emotions, reactions, and internal dialogue.

Common types of negative thinking include:

- **Catastrophizing**: Believing that the worst possible outcome will happen (e.g., "If I fail this test, my whole future is ruined").
- **All-or-nothing thinking**: Seeing situations in extremes, with no middle ground (e.g., "I'm either perfect or I'm a failure").

- **Overgeneralization**: Drawing broad conclusions based on one specific event (e.g., "I didn't get the job; I'll never find a job").
- **Mind reading**: Assuming you know what others are thinking, often in a negative light (e.g., "They think I'm incompetent").
- **Personalization**: Blaming yourself for events outside your control (e.g., "My friend is upset because of something I did").

2. Challenging the Negative Thoughts

Once you've identified a negative thought, the next step is to **challenge its accuracy**. Often, our negative thoughts are exaggerated or based on inaccurate assumptions. In this phase, CBT teaches individuals to assess the validity of their thoughts by asking critical questions.

Some common questions to ask when challenging a negative thought include:

- **Is this thought based on facts or assumptions?**
- **What evidence do I have to support this thought?**
- **Is there any evidence that contradicts this thought?**
- **What would I say to a friend who had this thought?**
- **What is the likelihood of this worst-case scenario happening?**
- **Is there another way to view this situation?**

For example, if you're thinking, "I'll never be successful," you might ask yourself:

- "What evidence do I have that I'm not successful?"
- "Have I experienced successes in my life, no matter how small?"
- "What would I tell a friend who had this same thought?"

This process encourages you to objectively analyze the thought, which often leads to discovering that it's less accurate or extreme than initially perceived.

3. Generating Alternative, Balanced Thoughts

After challenging a negative thought, the next step is to create a more **balanced** or **realistic** thought. This doesn't mean replacing negative thoughts with overly optimistic or unrealistic ones, but rather aiming for a more grounded and evidence-based perspective.

For example:

- If your original thought was "I'm going to fail this presentation," a balanced alternative could be "I've prepared well for this presentation, and even if I make a mistake, I can handle it."
- If you were thinking "I always mess up in social situations," you might reframe it to "Sometimes I feel awkward in social situations, but I can learn from those experiences and improve."

The goal is not to deny or dismiss the negative thoughts but to shift them toward more realistic, constructive alternatives that are based on evidence.

4. Examining the Impact of Reframing

Reframing negative thoughts is not just about changing what you think—it's also about changing how you **feel** and **behave** in response to those thoughts. Once a negative thought is reframed, you can observe the impact it has on your emotional state and actions. This process helps you develop new, healthier patterns of thinking that are less prone to emotional distress.

For example, after reframing a thought, you might notice:

- A reduction in anxiety or worry
- An increase in confidence or self-efficacy
- A decrease in avoidance behaviors (e.g., procrastination or withdrawing from social situations)
- Improved mood and emotional regulation

By consistently practicing the skill of reframing negative thoughts, individuals begin to retrain their thinking patterns and reduce their susceptibility to anxiety, depression, and other mental health challenges.

5. Using Thought Records to Track and Reframe Negative Thoughts

To help with the process of identifying and reframing negative thoughts, CBT often incorporates the use of **thought records**. These are worksheets or journals that allow individuals to document their negative thoughts, evaluate the evidence for and against them, and create more balanced alternatives. A typical thought record includes the following components:

1. **Situation**: What event triggered the negative thought?
2. **Negative Thought**: What was the automatic thought you had in response to the situation?
3. **Emotions**: What emotions did you feel as a result of the negative thought (e.g., anxiety, sadness, anger)?
4. **Evidence For the Thought**: What evidence supports the negative thought?
5. **Evidence Against the Thought**: What evidence contradicts the negative thought?
6. **Balanced Thought**: What is a more balanced, realistic thought you can adopt?
7. **Emotional Rating**: After reframing the thought, how do you feel now? Rate the intensity of your emotions again to see if it has changed.

This process allows you to track your cognitive distortions and better understand how to challenge them over time.

Practical Examples of Reframing Negative Thoughts

1. **Example 1: Overcoming Self-Doubt**
    - **Negative Thought**: "I'm not good enough for this job, and I'll never succeed."
    - **Challenging the Thought**: "What evidence do I have that I'm not good enough? I've been hired for

this position, and I have the necessary skills and experience."
- **Balanced Thought**: "I may have doubts, but I've succeeded in similar situations before, and I can ask for support when needed."
- **Reframed Emotion**: Reduced anxiety, increased confidence.

2. **Example 2: Managing Social Anxiety**
   - **Negative Thought**: "Everyone will judge me at this party. I'll make a fool of myself."
   - **Challenging the Thought**: "What makes me think everyone will judge me? I've been to social events before without incident, and people are usually focused on themselves."
   - **Balanced Thought**: "I might feel nervous, but I'm not the center of attention. Most people are just there to enjoy themselves."
   - **Reframed Emotion**: Reduced anxiety, increased comfort in social settings.

3. **Example 3: Dealing with Perfectionism**
   - **Negative Thought**: "If I don't get everything perfect, I'm a failure."
   - **Challenging the Thought**: "What's the evidence for this? I've been praised for my efforts, even when things weren't perfect. Nobody expects perfection."

Chapter 6: Positive Psychology for Anxiety

Positive Psychology and Its Role in Managing Anxiety

Positive psychology is a relatively modern branch of psychology that focuses on what makes life worth living—emphasizing strengths, resilience, and well-being rather than just treating mental illness. Unlike traditional approaches that primarily aim to alleviate suffering, positive psychology shifts the focus to enhancing positive emotions, fostering personal growth, and cultivating a sense of meaning and purpose. This approach can be particularly beneficial for individuals suffering from anxiety, offering practical tools and strategies that help them not only manage their symptoms but also build a greater sense of fulfillment and life satisfaction.

In this chapter, we will explore how positive psychology can be used to manage and even reduce anxiety. By focusing on strengths, cultivating gratitude, fostering optimism, and nurturing meaningful relationships, positive psychology provides a framework for creating a life that feels more grounded, resilient, and joyful—despite the challenges of anxiety.

Understanding Positive Psychology

Positive psychology emerged in the late 1990s, largely thanks to the work of psychologists such as **Martin Seligman**, who proposed a shift in focus from pathology (disease and disorders) to a more holistic view of human flourishing. According to Seligman, traditional psychology had concentrated too much on fixing what was broken, rather than enhancing what is already good in life. Positive psychology aims to answer questions like:

- **What makes life worth living?**
- **How can we cultivate more joy, peace, and resilience?**
- **How can people thrive in the face of adversity?**
- **How can we nurture our psychological and emotional well-being?**

Rather than focusing solely on the absence of anxiety or depression, positive psychology emphasizes developing the internal resources—such as hope, gratitude, and self-compassion—that can help individuals live meaningful, satisfying lives.

How Positive Psychology Helps People Suffering from Anxiety

While anxiety can feel overwhelming, it's important to recognize that anxiety is a natural response to perceived threats. Positive psychology doesn't dismiss the presence of anxiety; instead, it encourages individuals to shift their focus to cultivating positive emotions, building resilience, and strengthening coping mechanisms. This shift in focus can help reduce the intensity of anxious feelings and promote mental well-being.

Let's explore several key principles of positive psychology and how they can be applied to help manage anxiety:

1. Cultivating Positive Emotions

Positive emotions—such as joy, gratitude, love, and serenity—play a crucial role in well-being. People with high levels of positive emotion experience better mental health, including reduced symptoms of anxiety. Positive psychology encourages people to actively seek out and savor positive experiences, which can counterbalance the overwhelming nature of anxiety.

Strategies:

- **Savoring**: Take the time to savor small, pleasant moments in daily life. Whether it's enjoying a warm cup of coffee, listening to music, or appreciating a beautiful sunset, focusing on the positive aspects of your day can shift your perspective and help alleviate anxiety.
- **Gratitude Practice**: Keeping a gratitude journal is one of the simplest ways to boost positive emotions. By writing down things you're thankful for each day, you train your brain to notice the good things in life, which can reduce the focus on negative or anxiety-provoking thoughts.

Example:

- Start or end each day by writing down three things you're grateful for. They don't have to be big, but the act of recognizing the good in your life helps retrain your brain to focus on positive aspects, reducing anxiety's hold.

2. Strengthening Resilience

Anxiety often arises from feelings of powerlessness or fear of the future. Positive psychology emphasizes the importance of building **resilience**—the ability to bounce back from adversity. Resilience doesn't mean never feeling anxious or fearful; it means developing the inner strength to face and navigate life's challenges without becoming overwhelmed.

Strategies:

- **Building Psychological Flexibility**: Resilience involves being able to adapt to changing situations. Learning to tolerate uncertainty, which is often a key trigger for anxiety, can help individuals cope with difficult emotions more effectively.
- **Developing Optimism**: Positive psychology teaches people to cultivate optimism by reframing negative experiences and focusing on solutions rather than problems. For example, rather than thinking "This situation will never improve," try thinking "This situation is tough, but I can learn from it and grow."

Example:

- Engage in **cognitive reframing** to change the way you interpret anxious thoughts. Instead of thinking "I can't handle this," shift to "I've dealt with challenges before, and I can manage this too."

3. Fostering Meaning and Purpose

A sense of **meaning** and **purpose** in life can protect against the negative impacts of anxiety. People who feel that their lives have purpose are more likely to experience satisfaction and well-being. Positive psychology encourages individuals to connect with their values and passions, which can provide a sense of direction and fulfillment.

Strategies:

- **Identify Personal Values**: Spend time reflecting on what is most important to you—whether it's family, creativity, personal growth, or helping others. Aligning your daily actions with these values can help reduce feelings of anxiety by fostering a sense of control and purpose.
- **Engage in Meaningful Activities**: Spend time doing activities that align with your values and bring you joy. Whether it's volunteer work, creative expression, or spending quality time with loved ones, engaging in meaningful pursuits can act as a buffer against anxious thoughts and feelings.

Example:

- Reflect on a time when you felt particularly connected to your values or passions. It might have been a volunteer experience, a creative project, or an activity that felt deeply fulfilling. Focus on how those moments brought peace and perspective, and aim to incorporate similar activities into your routine.

4. Building Strengths and Self-Compassion

People who focus on developing their personal strengths are better equipped to manage life's difficulties, including anxiety. Positive psychology emphasizes identifying and leveraging your strengths—whether they are in creativity, leadership, humor, or kindness—to navigate challenges with confidence.

Strategies:

- **Strengths Assessment**: Take a strengths assessment, such as the **VIA Survey of Character Strengths**, to identify your unique strengths. Reflect on how you can use these strengths to cope with anxiety.
- **Self-Compassion**: A key principle of positive psychology is the cultivation of **self-compassion**—treating yourself with the same kindness and understanding that you would offer a close friend. Anxiety often triggers self-criticism, which exacerbates stress. Learning to be

compassionate toward yourself helps break the cycle of negative thinking.

Example:

- If you're feeling anxious about a work presentation, remind yourself of the strengths you have in communication or problem-solving. Treat yourself with compassion by acknowledging that it's okay to feel nervous, and that you are doing your best.

5. Social Connections and Support

Positive psychology emphasizes the importance of **social relationships** in fostering well-being. Strong, supportive relationships are a buffer against anxiety and can help provide perspective and emotional comfort in times of stress.

Strategies:

- **Nurture Relationships**: Spend quality time with friends and family who make you feel supported and understood. Social connections help reduce feelings of isolation and fear that often accompany anxiety.
- **Give and Receive Support**: Don't hesitate to seek support from others when needed. Equally important is offering support to those around you. Helping others fosters a sense of purpose and connection, reducing anxiety and promoting emotional well-being.

Example:

- When anxiety strikes, reach out to a trusted friend or family member to share how you're feeling. Talking about your experience can provide emotional relief and help you gain a different perspective on your concerns.

Challenging Negative Thoughts Using Positive Psychology

One of the key principles of positive psychology is the ability to shift focus from negative thinking patterns toward more positive, constructive ways of thinking. While negative thoughts and feelings are a natural part of human experience, they can become particularly overwhelming for those struggling with anxiety. Positive psychology offers effective strategies for challenging and transforming negative thoughts, fostering a more optimistic and balanced outlook on life.

In this section, we will explore techniques grounded in positive psychology that can help you challenge and reframe negative thoughts. By practicing these methods, you can reduce the impact of anxiety-provoking thoughts and build a more resilient, positive mindset.

1. Identifying and Interrupting Negative Thought Patterns

The first step in challenging negative thoughts is becoming aware of them. Often, negative thoughts arise automatically, leading to a cascade of emotional distress and anxious feelings. Positive psychology encourages the development of **mindfulness**—the practice of noticing thoughts without judgment. By observing your thoughts, you can begin to identify patterns of negativity, self-doubt, and fear that may be fueling your anxiety.

Strategies:

- **Mindfulness Practice**: Take a few minutes each day to practice mindfulness meditation. Focus on your breath, observe any thoughts that arise, and acknowledge them without judgment. As you observe your thoughts, notice if they are negative or unhelpful.
- **Thought Stopping**: When you notice a negative thought, mentally say "Stop!" and redirect your attention to something more positive or neutral. This simple technique helps disrupt the automatic flow of negative thinking and provides space for a more balanced response.

Example:
If you have the thought, "I'm going to fail at this presentation," take a moment to notice that thought, pause, and mentally say "Stop." Then, challenge that thought by asking yourself, "What evidence do I have that supports this?" and "What evidence contradicts this?"

Reframing negative thoughts is a core technique in positive psychology. It involves taking a negative thought or belief and replacing it with a more balanced or positive one. This doesn't mean ignoring negative feelings but rather viewing them through a more realistic lens. Reframing helps to shift your perspective and reduces the emotional charge associated with the negative thought.

Strategies:

- **The 3 Ps of Reframing**: When you catch yourself engaging in negative thinking, ask yourself:
    1. **Personalization**: Is this thought something I am taking too personally? For example, "I must have done something wrong" could be reframed to "I made a mistake, but everyone makes mistakes."
    2. **Permanence**: Is this feeling permanent, or is it temporary? For example, "This anxiety will never go away" can be reframed to "I'm anxious now, but this feeling will pass with time."
    3. **Pervasiveness**: Is this thought affecting all areas of my life? For example, "I can never handle anything" can be reframed to "I struggled with this situation, but I have handled challenges in the past and can learn from this."
- **Best Possible Self Exercise**: Imagine your best possible future—what would life look like if everything went as well as it possibly could? Visualizing positive

outcomes can shift your focus away from anxiety-driven fears to the potential for success and fulfillment.

Example: If you have a thought like "I always mess things up," reframe it with a more balanced thought: "I've made mistakes, but I have learned from them and improved each time."

3. Gratitude Practice

Gratitude is one of the most powerful tools in positive psychology for shifting negative thinking patterns. When you're feeling anxious or overwhelmed, it's easy to focus on everything that could go wrong. However, by consciously practicing gratitude, you can redirect your focus to the positive aspects of your life, fostering feelings of contentment and reducing anxiety.

Strategies:

- **Gratitude Journal**: Keep a gratitude journal where you write down three things you are grateful for each day. This simple practice helps you focus on the positive, rather than dwelling on anxiety-provoking thoughts.
- **Gratitude Meditation**: Set aside time each day to meditate on the things you are grateful for. This can be as simple as focusing on the warmth of the sun, your health, your loved ones, or accomplishments, no matter how small.

Example:
If you're feeling anxious about a challenging situation, such as an upcoming test or presentation, take a moment to list things you are grateful for in your life—your support system, the opportunity to grow, your skills, and even the ability to work through discomfort. This helps ground you in the present moment and reduces the impact of anxiety.

4. Rewriting Your Story: Narrative Psychology

Narrative psychology is an aspect of positive psychology that focuses on the stories we tell ourselves about our lives. These personal narratives shape our identity and influence how we interpret events and experiences. By recognizing the negative stories we tell about ourselves and rewriting them in a more empowering way, we can reduce anxiety and increase our sense of agency and control.

Strategies:

- **Rewriting Your Narrative**: When you notice negative thoughts about yourself, ask yourself, "What's the story I'm telling myself about this situation?" For example, if you're anxious about a presentation, the story might be "I'm terrible at speaking in public, and I'm going to embarrass myself." To rewrite this story, consider how you can view it from a different angle. For instance, "Public speaking is challenging for me, but I've prepared and I can handle this."

- **Self-Compassionate Reframing**: Instead of seeing yourself as a failure when things go wrong, reframe the story to focus on your resilience and capacity for growth. For example, "I didn't do as well as I hoped, but I can learn from this experience and improve next time."

Example:
If you often have the thought "I'm not good enough," rewrite that story to "I am constantly learning and growing, and I have the ability to succeed, even when things don't go perfectly."

5. Fostering Optimism

Optimism is a foundational aspect of positive psychology. It involves the ability to see challenges as temporary and specific, rather than permanent and pervasive. Optimism can significantly reduce anxiety by helping individuals focus on potential solutions and positive outcomes instead of fixating on worst-case scenarios.

Strategies:

- **Pessimism vs. Optimism Exercise**: When you catch yourself thinking negatively, ask yourself how an optimistic person would perceive the same situation. For example, if you are worried about an upcoming job interview, an optimistic thought might be, "I've prepared, I have the skills, and I'm doing my best. Even if I don't get this job, I'll find another opportunity."

- **Challenge Catastrophic Thinking**: Anxiety often involves catastrophic thinking, where we imagine the worst possible outcomes. Challenge this by asking yourself, "What's the worst that could happen, and how likely is it?" Then, remind yourself of the many possible positive outcomes.

Example:
If you're thinking "I can't handle this situation," counter it with an optimistic thought such as "I've faced challenges before, and I have the strength and tools to manage this one as well."

PERMA in Positive Psychology: A Framework for Flourishing

The **PERMA model** is one of the most influential frameworks in positive psychology, developed by psychologist **Martin Seligman** as a way to understand and enhance well-being. Unlike traditional models of mental health that focus on alleviating dysfunction, the PERMA model emphasizes **what makes life worth living** and identifies five key elements that contribute to a flourishing life. These five elements—**Positive Emotion, Engagement, Relationships, Meaning,** and **Accomplishment**—are all essential components of well-being and can be cultivated through specific practices to improve mental health, including the management of anxiety.

In this section, we'll explore the **PERMA model** in depth, breaking down each element and offering practical ways to apply them to your life, particularly in managing anxiety and promoting emotional well-being.

1. Positive Emotion

Positive Emotion refers to the experience of pleasant feelings such as joy, gratitude, contentment, and hope. While negative emotions like anxiety, fear, and sadness are natural and valid, fostering more positive emotions can counterbalance their effects and help build resilience. Experiencing positive emotions also improves physical health, strengthens relationships, and supports better decision-making.

How Positive Emotions Help with Anxiety:

- **Counteracting Negative Bias**: Anxiety often leads to negative thinking, where we focus on potential threats or worst-case scenarios. Experiencing positive emotions helps counteract this negativity by broadening our perspective and making it easier to see opportunities and solutions.
- **Promoting Relaxation**: Positive emotions like joy and gratitude trigger the release of neurochemicals like dopamine and serotonin, which help lower stress levels and reduce anxiety.

- **Gratitude Practice**: Writing down things you're grateful for every day can help shift your focus away from anxious thoughts and towards the positives in your life.
- **Pleasant Activities**: Engage in activities that make you feel good, whether it's a hobby, a walk in nature, or spending time with friends. The more positive experiences you have, the more they can offset feelings of anxiety.

Example:
Try keeping a **gratitude journal**, where you jot down three things you are thankful for every day. This helps reinforce positive thinking and can be particularly useful during times of high anxiety.

2. Engagement

Engagement is the state of being fully immersed in an activity—where time seems to stand still, and you are completely absorbed in the task at hand. This is often referred to as the experience of being in **"flow."** When you are deeply engaged in something, you are not focused on your worries or anxious thoughts; instead, you are present and enjoying the moment.

- **Distraction from Worries**: Engaging in meaningful activities or hobbies can help distract from the constant stream of anxious thoughts.
- **Building Competence**: Being engaged in tasks where you can develop your skills enhances your sense of competence and control, which can help reduce feelings of helplessness often associated with anxiety.
- **Enhancing Self-Esteem**: Flow activities boost self-confidence by allowing you to experience success and mastery, which in turn helps mitigate anxious thoughts.

Practical Strategies:

- **Find Your Flow**: Identify activities that deeply engage you—whether it's painting, solving puzzles, exercising, or playing music. These are your "flow" activities that will allow you to escape from anxious thoughts and immerse yourself in something enjoyable and productive.
- **Mindful Engagement**: Practicing mindfulness during everyday tasks can help you become more engaged and present. Whether you are washing dishes, walking, or working, focus on the sensory details of the activity and try to become absorbed in the moment.

Example:
If you're feeling anxious, engage in a creative activity, such as writing, drawing, or playing a musical instrument. By focusing your attention on the task, you naturally shift away from your worries and into a state of deep engagement.

3. Relationships

Positive relationships are essential for well-being. Human beings are social creatures, and the quality of our relationships with others plays a huge role in our overall happiness and mental health. Having supportive, loving, and meaningful connections with friends, family, and colleagues helps reduce stress and anxiety, boosts self-esteem, and promotes a sense of belonging.

How Relationships Help with Anxiety:

- **Social Support**: During times of anxiety, turning to a supportive friend or loved one can provide comfort, reassurance, and perspective. Feeling connected to others helps buffer the effects of anxiety.
- **Sense of Belonging**: Healthy relationships create a sense of belonging and security, which can diminish feelings of isolation or loneliness that often accompany anxiety.
- **Emotional Validation**: Sharing your thoughts and feelings with others helps validate your emotions and can give you new insights, which can help reduce anxious rumination.

Practical Strategies:

- **Invest in Relationships**: Take time to nurture your closest relationships. Regularly check in with family and

friends, spend time together, and engage in open, supportive conversations.
- **Seek Professional Support**: If you feel comfortable, consider seeking support from a therapist or counselor. They provide a safe, non-judgmental space to discuss your anxiety and help you develop strategies to manage it.

Example:
If you're feeling anxious, reach out to a trusted friend or family member for support. Sometimes just talking things through with someone who listens can provide tremendous relief.

4. Meaning

Meaning refers to having a sense of purpose or belonging in life. It's about feeling that your life has significance, that your actions are aligned with your values, and that you contribute to something greater than yourself. When you have a strong sense of meaning, you feel more motivated, resilient, and capable of handling challenges, including anxiety.

How Meaning Helps with Anxiety:
- **Shifting Focus**: Anxiety often arises when we focus on ourselves or the future in a fearful way. Having a sense of meaning shifts the focus outward—towards something larger, such as your community, your work, or your values—which can help diminish anxiety.

- **Building Resilience**: People with a sense of meaning are better able to face adversity with strength and perseverance because they feel their struggles serve a greater purpose.
- **Enhancing Well-being**: Meaningful activities—whether it's helping others, pursuing a passion, or following your values—can increase life satisfaction and reduce anxiety.

Practical Strategies:

- **Clarify Your Values**: Take some time to reflect on what matters most to you—what are your core values? Whether it's family, creativity, community, or personal growth, identifying these values can help you find more meaning in your daily life.
- **Engage in Purposeful Work**: Find ways to engage in work or activities that are aligned with your values. Volunteering, mentoring, or creating something meaningful can give you a sense of purpose and reduce feelings of anxiety.

Example:
If you feel overwhelmed by anxiety, consider volunteering or helping someone in need. Giving back to others can remind you that your actions have meaning and contribute to the well-being of others.

5. Accomplishment

The final element of the PERMA model is **Accomplishment**—the sense of achieving goals, mastering challenges, and reaching milestones. This element emphasizes the importance of progress and success, which boost self-esteem, increase motivation, and contribute to a sense of competence.

How Accomplishment Helps with Anxiety:

- **Building Confidence**: Accomplishing small goals, even if they seem insignificant, reinforces your belief in your ability to handle challenges and cope with anxiety.
- **Motivating Action**: Setting and achieving goals helps create momentum, encouraging you to take action rather than getting stuck in worry and fear.
- **Creating a Sense of Mastery**: Achieving a goal, big or small, provides a tangible sense of mastery, which can reduce feelings of helplessness often linked to anxiety.

Practical Strategies:

- **Set Small, Achievable Goals**: Break down larger tasks into smaller, manageable steps. Celebrate each success along the way to reinforce your sense of accomplishment.
- **Track Progress**: Keep a journal or use an app to track your progress toward your goals. Reflecting on your achievements can provide motivation and boost your self-esteem.

Example:
If you feel anxious about a large task, such as preparing for a presentation, break it down into smaller steps—researching, creating slides, rehearsing. Celebrate each accomplishment along the way to build confidence and reduce anxiety.

The **PERMA model** offers a comprehensive framework for improving well-being and managing anxiety. By focusing on Positive Emotion, Engagement, Relationships, Meaning, and Accomplishment, individuals can create a life that promotes resilience, happiness, and fulfillment, even in the face of anxiety. Incorporating the principles of positive psychology into your daily routine can help you build the inner resources to handle anxiety more effectively, creating a greater sense of peace and satisfaction in your life.

Chapter 7: Mindfulness Based Stress Reduction (MBSR)

In a world filled with constant demands, rapid changes, and unrelenting pressures, stress has become a common experience for many. For those grappling with anxiety, stress can feel even more overwhelming, feeding into cycles of worry, fear, and physical tension. **Mindfulness-Based Stress Reduction (MBSR)** offers a powerful, evidence-based approach to managing stress and anxiety, promoting a sense of calm, balance, and self-awareness.

Developed in the late 1970s by Dr. **Jon Kabat-Zinn** at the University of Massachusetts Medical School, MBSR is an eight-week program designed to help individuals cultivate mindfulness as a tool to cope with stress, pain, and difficult emotions. Rooted in ancient meditative practices and combined with modern psychological insights, MBSR has been extensively researched and proven effective in reducing symptoms of anxiety, depression, and chronic stress.

At its core, MBSR is about living in the present moment. It teaches us to respond to life's challenges with clarity and intention rather than reacting impulsively or being overwhelmed by negative thoughts and emotions. By focusing attention on the "here and now," MBSR helps break the cycle of rumination and anticipatory fear that often accompanies anxiety.

In this chapter, we will explore the foundations of Mindfulness-Based Stress Reduction, how it works, and why it has become one of the most respected and widely practiced methods for stress and anxiety management. You will learn about the principles of mindfulness, the science behind MBSR, and practical techniques you can incorporate into your daily life to cultivate peace and resilience in the face of stress.

Mindfulness, as taught through MBSR, is not just a practice but a way of being—a gentle, non-judgmental awareness of the present moment that allows us to approach life's challenges with greater ease and compassion. Let's dive into the transformative potential of mindfulness and discover how MBSR can empower you to navigate life with a greater sense of calm and confidence.

Understanding MBSR and Its Benefits for Anxiety and Panic Disorder

Mindfulness-Based Stress Reduction (MBSR) is a structured program that combines mindfulness meditation and gentle yoga to enhance self-awareness and manage stress. For individuals experiencing anxiety or panic disorders, MBSR offers practical tools to navigate distressing emotions and physical sensations with greater control and calmness.

At its heart, MBSR emphasizes **mindful awareness**—paying attention to the present moment with an attitude of curiosity, openness, and non-judgment. For those with anxiety, this approach can be transformative. Anxiety often pulls the mind into the past, replaying regrets, or into the future, anticipating worst-case scenarios. MBSR helps ground individuals in the **here and now**, breaking the cycle of catastrophic thinking and physical tension.

How MBSR Works

MBSR is built on regular mindfulness practices that include:

1. **Mindful Breathing**: Observing the breath as it flows in and out, anchoring attention to the present moment.
2. **Body Scan**: Bringing attention to different parts of the body to cultivate awareness and release tension.
3. **Mindful Movement**: Incorporating gentle yoga or stretching to connect the mind and body.
4. **Sitting Meditation**: Focusing on thoughts, sensations, or sounds while practicing non-reactivity.

Participants of an MBSR program typically meet for weekly group sessions and engage in daily mindfulness practices at home. These practices help develop a **heightened awareness of thoughts, emotions, and physical sensations**, which can disrupt automatic reactions to stress and foster healthier responses.

Benefits of MBSR for Anxiety and Panic Disorder

1. Breaking the Fight-or-Flight Cycle

For individuals with anxiety or panic disorder, the body often remains stuck in a **fight-or-flight response**, even in the absence of real danger. MBSR helps retrain the nervous system by promoting relaxation and activating the

parasympathetic nervous system, which restores balance and reduces physical symptoms of anxiety such as rapid heart rate, sweating, and shortness of breath.

2. Cultivating Non-Judgmental Awareness

Anxiety thrives on self-criticism and resistance to uncomfortable emotions. MBSR teaches individuals to **accept their thoughts and feelings without judgment**, creating a sense of psychological space. This approach reduces the power of anxious thoughts, making them less overwhelming.

3. Reducing Avoidance Behaviors

People with anxiety or panic often avoid situations or triggers that they perceive as threatening. This avoidance can reinforce fear and limit daily functioning. MBSR encourages a mindful approach to difficult situations, helping individuals face their fears with **greater courage and presence**, leading to long-term desensitization and resilience.

4. Enhancing Emotional Regulation

Mindfulness practice helps individuals become more aware of their emotional states and develop healthier coping mechanisms. Over time, this leads to **better control over emotional reactions** and reduces the intensity of anxious episodes.

Anxiety often disrupts sleep, creating a vicious cycle where lack of rest exacerbates stress. MBSR practices, particularly body scans and mindful breathing, help calm the mind and body, promoting deeper and more restful sleep.

6. Boosting Self-Compassion

MBSR fosters self-compassion—a critical tool for reducing the shame and self-blame that often accompany anxiety disorders. By practicing kindness towards themselves, individuals can break free from negative self-talk and build a more supportive inner dialogue.

7. Building Long-Term Resilience

The skills learned in MBSR extend beyond the eight-week program. Regular mindfulness practice reshapes how individuals respond to stress, creating a lasting sense of resilience and emotional balance.

Scientific Evidence Supporting MBSR

Extensive research has demonstrated the effectiveness of MBSR in managing anxiety and panic disorders. Studies have shown that:

- MBSR significantly reduces symptoms of **generalized anxiety disorder (GAD)** by improving emotional regulation and stress tolerance.
- It is as effective as cognitive-behavioral therapy (CBT) for many individuals with anxiety disorders.

- Regular mindfulness practice leads to **structural changes in the brain**, such as increased gray matter density in areas responsible for emotion regulation and decreased activity in the amygdala, which is hyperactive in individuals with anxiety.

Case Example

Imagine someone experiencing frequent panic attacks. Before practicing MBSR, their typical response might involve avoiding triggers, hyperventilating, or feeling trapped by fear. After completing an MBSR program, they learn to recognize the early signs of a panic attack, use mindful breathing to anchor themselves, and allow the sensations to pass without resistance. Over time, the intensity and frequency of their panic attacks decrease, and they feel more empowered to face previously feared situations.

How to Get Started with MBSR

If you're interested in exploring MBSR:

1. **Join a Program**: Look for an MBSR course in your area or online, guided by a trained instructor.
2. **Practice Daily**: Begin incorporating mindfulness exercises into your routine, such as a 10-minute body scan or mindful breathing session.
3. **Be Patient**: MBSR is not a quick fix but a gradual process that yields profound, long-lasting benefits with consistent practice.

Challenging Negative Thoughts Using MBSR

One of the most powerful tools provided by **Mindfulness-Based Stress Reduction (MBSR)** is its ability to help individuals recognize, understand, and challenge their negative thought patterns. Anxiety often thrives on automatic negative thoughts (ANTs), which are habitual and distorted ways of thinking that reinforce fear, self-doubt, and worry. By cultivating mindfulness, MBSR enables individuals to observe these thoughts without being consumed by them, creating space for a more balanced and objective perspective.

How MBSR Helps Address Negative Thoughts

1. Observing Without Judgment

Mindfulness encourages a practice of **non-judgmental observation**. Instead of reacting to negative thoughts or trying to suppress them, MBSR teaches you to simply notice them as mental events, much like watching clouds pass in the sky. This practice creates distance between you and your thoughts, reducing their emotional impact.

For example:
A thought such as *"I'm not good enough"* can be acknowledged as just a thought, not an absolute truth. By labeling it as *"self-doubt"* or *"anxiety speaking,"* you gain power over it.

2. Breaking the Cycle of Rumination

Negative thoughts often trigger a cycle of rumination, where the mind replays worries or fears in a loop. MBSR interrupts this process by shifting your attention back to the present moment. Through mindful breathing or grounding techniques, you can redirect your focus from unproductive thinking to your immediate experience, effectively breaking the hold of rumination.

For example:
When your mind fixates on *"What if everything goes wrong?"* mindfulness practice helps you return to *"What is happening right now?"*

3. Cultivating Self-Compassion

Negative thoughts are frequently fueled by self-criticism, which can exacerbate anxiety. MBSR integrates **self-compassion practices** that encourage kindness and understanding toward yourself, particularly during moments of struggle. When faced with a harsh inner critic, MBSR invites you to respond as you would to a close friend—with warmth and reassurance.

For example:
Instead of saying, *"I'm such a failure for feeling this way,"* you

might say, *"It's okay to feel anxious right now. I'm doing the best I can."*

4. Using the Body Scan to Identify Emotional Patterns

Negative thoughts often manifest as physical sensations, such as tightness in the chest or tension in the shoulders. The **body scan**, a core MBSR practice, helps you tune into these sensations with curiosity and acceptance. By connecting your mental and physical experiences, you can begin to recognize how negative thoughts influence your body and vice versa.

For example:
During a body scan, you may notice that feelings of anxiety are linked to shallow breathing or a clenched jaw. Awareness of these patterns allows you to release tension and address the underlying thoughts with greater clarity.

5. Reframing Through Mindful Awareness

Mindfulness encourages reframing—seeing negative thoughts through a more neutral or positive lens. This isn't about forcing optimism but about recognizing alternative perspectives. By staying present, you can challenge automatic assumptions and replace them with more constructive thoughts.

For example:
Instead of thinking, *"I'll never succeed,"* mindfulness might allow you to recognize, *"I'm feeling discouraged right now, but that doesn't mean I won't succeed in the future."*

Practical MBSR Exercises to Challenge Negative Thoughts

1. **Thought Labeling**:
   When a negative thought arises, give it a neutral label, such as *"worry," "fear,"* or *"self-doubt."* This practice creates psychological distance and reduces the thought's power.
   - Example: A thought like *"I'm going to fail at this presentation"* can be labeled as *"fear of failure."*
2. **RAIN Technique**:
   Acknowledge and process negative thoughts using the **RAIN** acronym:
   - **R**ecognize the thought.
   - **A**ccept it without judgment.
   - **I**nvestigate its origins and emotions.
   - **N**urture yourself with kindness.
   - Example: Recognize that you're feeling anxious, accept that it's okay to feel this way, investigate why this moment feels threatening, and nurture yourself with words like, *"This is temporary, and I can handle it."*

3. **Three-Minute Breathing Space**:
   Use this quick mindfulness exercise when negative thoughts feel overwhelming:
   - **Step 1**: Acknowledge what you're thinking and feeling.
   - **Step 2**: Focus on your breath, grounding yourself in the present moment.
   - **Step 3**: Expand your awareness to your body and environment, creating a broader perspective.
4. **Gratitude Mindfulness**:
   When consumed by negativity, pause and bring to mind three things you're grateful for in that moment. This practice shifts your focus from what's wrong to what's right.

The Long-Term Impact of MBSR on Negative Thoughts

With consistent practice, MBSR can transform your relationship with negative thoughts. Rather than seeing them as enemies to fight or truths to believe, you begin to view them as fleeting mental events that do not define you. Over time, this shift fosters greater resilience, emotional balance, and confidence in your ability to face life's challenges.

By combining mindfulness with kindness, awareness, and acceptance, MBSR offers a gentle yet powerful way to challenge and reduce the influence of negative thoughts, paving the way for greater peace and clarity in your life.

Chapter 8: Lifestyle Changes for Better Mental Health

Adopting lifestyle changes to improve mental health is not a one-size-fits-all process—it's a deeply personal journey. While there is no universal roadmap, the key to success lies in finding small, achievable shifts that resonate with your values, interests, and goals. These changes, though gradual, have the potential to create lasting, meaningful improvements in your mental well-being.

Lifestyle changes act as a foundation for mental health by promoting balance, resilience, and a sense of control in an unpredictable world. They provide tools to strengthen your body and mind, preparing you to better handle life's challenges. Unlike quick fixes or rigid self-improvement plans, sustainable lifestyle adjustments emphasize self-compassion, patience, and consistency.

The Holistic Approach to Mental Health

A holistic approach means looking beyond symptoms and addressing the root causes of mental health challenges. Lifestyle choices influence several factors tied to mental health, such as:

1. Brain Chemistry: Activities like exercise and proper nutrition influence neurotransmitters like serotonin, dopamine, and endorphins, which regulate mood.

2. Stress Regulation: Simple practices such as mindfulness, quality sleep, and reduced screen time lower the body's stress response, reducing cortisol levels.
3. Emotional Balance: Social connections, physical activity, and engaging in fulfilling hobbies cultivate a sense of joy, purpose, and belonging.
4. Cognitive Function: Adequate rest, physical activity, and nutrition sharpen focus, memory, and decision-making.

Why Lifestyle Changes Matter

Many aspects of daily life contribute to mental health in ways that are easy to overlook. Chronic stress, irregular sleep, poor diet, and lack of movement can gradually erode mental wellness. By addressing these factors, you can create an environment—both internally and externally—that supports growth, healing, and positivity.

Small Changes, Big Impact

The secret to successful lifestyle changes lies in starting small. Trying to completely overhaul your habits all at once can lead to frustration and burnout. Instead, focus on incremental steps:

- Swap one sugary snack for a nutritious alternative.
- Dedicate five minutes to mindful breathing each day.
- Take a ten-minute walk after dinner.

- Replace 15 minutes of screen time with journaling or reading before bed.

Over time, these small changes compound into significant results. They help build momentum and confidence, making it easier to incorporate additional habits.

The Role of Exercise in Reducing Anxiety

Exercise is one of the most effective, accessible, and natural ways to reduce anxiety. It not only improves physical health but also provides profound mental health benefits. Regular physical activity directly impacts the brain and body systems associated with stress and anxiety, helping individuals manage symptoms and build long-term resilience.

Whether it's a brisk walk, yoga session, or weightlifting at the gym, exercise engages the body and mind in ways that counteract the physiological and psychological mechanisms of anxiety.

The Science Behind Exercise and Anxiety Relief

1. Balancing Brain Chemistry

Exercise stimulates the release of neurotransmitters such as **serotonin, dopamine**, and **endorphins**, often called "feel-good" chemicals. These neurotransmitters help stabilize mood, alleviate stress, and create a sense of well-being.

Additionally, exercise can reduce the activity of the **amygdala**, the brain's fear center, which is hyperactive in individuals with anxiety. This results in decreased feelings of worry and a calmer mental state.

2. Regulating the Stress Response

Anxiety is often characterized by an overactive **fight-or-flight response**, leading to physical symptoms like rapid heartbeat, shallow breathing, and muscle tension. Exercise provides a controlled outlet for this energy, helping to discharge stress hormones like **cortisol** and lower the overall baseline of arousal.

For example:

- Aerobic activities like running or swimming reduce cortisol levels, promoting relaxation.
- Gentle exercises like yoga encourage parasympathetic activity, also known as the "rest-and-digest" response.

3. Building Resilience to Stress

Over time, regular physical activity helps the brain and body become more adaptable to stress. Exercise strengthens neural connections in areas like the **prefrontal cortex**, which is involved in decision-making and emotional regulation. This increased resilience means you're less likely to experience anxiety when faced with challenges.

Mental and Emotional Benefits of Exercise

1. Breaking the Cycle of Rumination

Anxiety often leads to rumination—repetitive, negative thought patterns that exacerbate distress. Engaging in physical activity redirects your focus to the present moment, interrupting these cycles. Activities like yoga or mindful walking further enhance this benefit by incorporating intentional breathing and mindfulness.

2. Improving Sleep

Exercise promotes better sleep quality, which is critical for managing anxiety. Physical activity helps regulate the body's natural circadian rhythm and reduces insomnia, allowing for restorative rest that enhances mood and cognitive function.

3. Boosting Self-Esteem

Meeting exercise goals, no matter how small, builds a sense of accomplishment and self-worth. For individuals struggling with anxiety, this boost in confidence can help counter feelings of helplessness or inadequacy.

4. Enhancing Social Connection

Group activities like team sports, dance classes, or walking groups foster social interaction, which is a powerful antidote to anxiety. These connections create a sense of belonging and support, reducing feelings of isolation.

Types of Exercise for Anxiety Relief

1. Cardio Exercise

Activities like running, cycling, swimming, or brisk walking are particularly effective for reducing anxiety. Aerobic exercise increases heart rate and stimulates the release of endorphins, often leading to what's known as a "runner's high."

2. Strength Training

Weightlifting and resistance exercises have been shown to lower anxiety symptoms, particularly by providing a sense of control and mastery. They also release endorphins and improve physical strength, which can boost self-confidence.

3. Yoga and Tai Chi

These practices combine physical movement with mindfulness, deep breathing, and body awareness. They are especially effective for reducing the physical tension associated with anxiety while promoting relaxation and inner peace.

4. Walking or Hiking

Even moderate-intensity activities like walking can have profound effects on mental health. Walking in nature, or **ecotherapy**, is particularly beneficial as it combines movement with exposure to calming natural environments. Walking meditations (via any tech device) suffice as well.

5. High-Intensity Interval Training (HIIT)

For individuals who enjoy more vigorous workouts, HIIT can offer rapid mood-boosting benefits. These short bursts of intense activity followed by rest periods can help burn off excess energy and stress.

Practical Tips for Incorporating Exercise

1. **Start Small**: If you're new to exercise, aim for just 10–15 minutes a day. Gradually increase the duration and intensity as you become more comfortable.
2. **Choose Enjoyable Activities**: Exercise doesn't have to mean going to the gym. Dancing, gardening, or playing with a pet can be equally beneficial.
3. **Incorporate Movement Into Your Day**: Take the stairs instead of the elevator, stretch during breaks, or go for a short walk after meals.
4. **Be Consistent**: Aim for regular activity, such as 3–5 sessions per week. Consistency is more important than intensity.

5. **Combine Exercise with Mindfulness**: Focus on your breathing, bodily sensations, or surroundings while exercising to maximize its calming effects.

Nutrition and Its Impact on Anxiety

The saying "you are what you eat" holds more truth than many realize, especially when it comes to mental health. The relationship between diet and anxiety is a growing area of research, revealing that the food we consume not only affects our physical health but also has a significant impact on brain function and emotional well-being.

A balanced, nutrient-rich diet can help regulate mood, reduce inflammation, and stabilize blood sugar levels—all of which play a role in managing anxiety. Conversely, poor eating habits, such as excessive sugar intake or skipping meals, can exacerbate anxiety symptoms and increase stress.

The Gut-Brain Connection

Central to understanding the relationship between nutrition and anxiety is the **gut-brain axis**, a communication system between the gastrointestinal tract and the brain. The gut is often referred to as the "second brain" because it produces neurotransmitters like serotonin, which influence mood and anxiety levels.

1. **Gut Microbiota**:
   The gut is home to trillions of microbes that play a crucial role in mental health. A diverse and balanced gut microbiome supports emotional resilience, while an imbalance (dysbiosis) can contribute to anxiety and depression.
2. **The Role of Inflammation**:
   Poor dietary choices can lead to chronic inflammation, which is linked to increased anxiety symptoms. Anti-inflammatory foods, such as those rich in omega-3 fatty acids, can help counteract this effect.

Key Nutrients for Reducing Anxiety

Certain nutrients are particularly beneficial for managing anxiety, as they support brain health, regulate stress hormones, and promote a sense of calm.

1. Omega-3 Fatty Acids

- Found in: Fatty fish (salmon, mackerel, sardines), chia seeds, walnuts, flaxseeds.
- Benefits: Omega-3s reduce inflammation and support brain function, improving mood and reducing anxiety symptoms.

2. Magnesium

- Found in: Leafy greens (spinach, kale), nuts (almonds, cashews), seeds, whole grains, avocados.

- Benefits: Magnesium helps regulate the body's stress response and promotes relaxation.

3. Vitamin B Complex

- Found in: Whole grains, eggs, dairy, leafy greens, legumes, poultry.
- Benefits: B vitamins, particularly B6 and B12, are essential for the production of neurotransmitters like serotonin and dopamine.

4. Probiotics

- Found in: Yogurt, kefir, sauerkraut, kimchi, miso, kombucha.
- Benefits: Probiotics support a healthy gut microbiome, which is crucial for regulating mood and reducing anxiety.

5. Tryptophan

- Found in: Turkey, chicken, eggs, cheese, nuts, seeds, bananas.
- Benefits: Tryptophan is an amino acid that helps the body produce serotonin, which promotes a sense of calm.

6. Complex Carbohydrates

- Found in: Whole grains, oats, quinoa, sweet potatoes, legumes.
- Benefits: These foods provide a steady source of energy, preventing blood sugar spikes that can trigger anxiety.

7. Antioxidants

- Found in: Berries, dark chocolate, green tea, colorful vegetables (bell peppers, carrots, broccoli).
- Benefits: Antioxidants protect the brain from oxidative stress, which can contribute to anxiety.
-

Foods to Limit or Avoid

While some foods can support mental health, others may exacerbate anxiety symptoms and should be consumed in moderation.

1. Caffeine

- Found in: Coffee, energy drinks, soda, chocolate.
- Why Limit: Caffeine stimulates the nervous system and can mimic or worsen anxiety symptoms like rapid heartbeat and restlessness.

2. Sugar and Refined Carbs

- Found in: Sugary snacks, white bread, pastries, soda.
- Why Limit: These foods cause blood sugar spikes and crashes, leading to mood swings and increased anxiety.

3. Alcohol

- Why Limit: Alcohol can temporarily reduce anxiety but often worsens symptoms over time by disrupting sleep and brain chemistry.

- **Processed food** Found in: Packaged snacks, fast food, frozen meals.
- Why Limit: These foods are often high in unhealthy fats, sugar, and salt, contributing to inflammation and poor gut health.

Practical Tips for Anxiety-Reducing Nutrition

1. **Eat Balanced Meals**: Aim for a mix of protein, healthy fats, and complex carbohydrates at each meal to keep blood sugar levels stable.
2. **Stay Hydrated**: Dehydration can cause irritability and fatigue, which may amplify anxiety.
3. **Plan Ahead**: Prepare healthy snacks and meals to avoid turning to processed or fast food when you're busy or stressed.
4. **Focus on Whole Foods**: Incorporate fresh, minimally processed ingredients into your diet for maximum nutrient density.
5. **Mindful Eating**: Pay attention to your hunger and fullness cues, savor your meals, and avoid distractions like screens while eating.
6. **Experiment with Probiotic Foods**: Incorporate fermented foods into your diet to support gut health and mood regulation.

Sleep is the foundation of physical and mental health, playing a crucial role in emotional regulation, cognitive function, and overall well-being. For individuals managing anxiety, quality sleep is especially vital, as insufficient rest can exacerbate symptoms and reduce resilience to stress.

Sleep hygiene refers to the habits, routines, and environmental factors that promote restful and restorative sleep. By understanding the relationship between anxiety and sleep and implementing strategies to improve sleep hygiene, individuals can enhance their ability to manage stress and foster a sense of calm.

The Relationship Between Anxiety and Sleep

Anxiety and sleep disturbances often form a vicious cycle. Anxiety can make it difficult to fall asleep or stay asleep, while lack of sleep amplifies feelings of worry and stress.

How Anxiety Disrupts Sleep

1. **Hyperarousal**: The heightened state of alertness associated with anxiety can prevent the mind and body from relaxing enough to sleep.
2. **Racing Thoughts**: Persistent worries or rumination can make it challenging to quiet the mind at bedtime.

Effects of Poor Sleep on Anxiety

1. **Increased Stress Response**: Sleep deprivation heightens the activity of the amygdala, the brain's fear center, making individuals more reactive to stress.
2. **Impaired Emotional Regulation**: Lack of sleep weakens the prefrontal cortex, the part of the brain responsible for managing emotions and rational thinking.
3. **Lowered Resilience**: Without adequate rest, coping mechanisms are less effective, leading to a greater sense of overwhelm.

Benefits of Good Sleep Hygiene for Anxiety

1. **Regulates Mood**: Quality sleep reduces irritability and promotes emotional balance.
2. **Enhances Cognitive Function**: A well-rested brain is better equipped to process information, solve problems, and focus on positive thoughts.
3. **Strengthens Coping Mechanisms**: Restorative sleep enhances resilience, making it easier to handle stress and anxiety triggers.
4. **Supports Physical Health**: Sleep reduces inflammation and strengthens the immune system, which can help minimize the physical impact of anxiety.

1. Establish a Consistent Sleep Schedule

- Go to bed and wake up at the same time every day, even on weekends.
- Consistency helps regulate your body's internal clock (circadian rhythm), making it easier to fall asleep and wake up feeling refreshed.

2. Create a Relaxing Bedtime Routine

- Develop calming rituals before bed, such as reading, meditating, or taking a warm bath.
- Avoid stimulating activities like work, intense exercise, or scrolling through social media close to bedtime.

3. Optimize Your Sleep Environment

- Keep your bedroom cool, dark, and quiet. Use blackout curtains, a fan, or white noise if needed.
- Invest in a comfortable mattress and pillows.
- Reserve your bed for sleep and intimacy only, avoiding work or screen time in bed.

4. Limit Stimulants and Substances

- Avoid caffeine, nicotine, and large meals in the hours leading up to bedtime.
- Be mindful of alcohol consumption, as it can disrupt sleep quality.

- Engage in relaxation exercises such as deep breathing, progressive muscle relaxation, or mindfulness meditation to calm your mind before sleep.
- Use apps or guided meditations designed to help you unwind.

6. Manage Worries and Racing Thoughts

- Keep a journal by your bedside to jot down worries or to-do lists before bed. This helps clear your mind for sleep.
- Try cognitive behavioral techniques, such as reframing negative thoughts, to reduce nighttime anxiety.

7. Limit Screen Time

- Turn off electronic devices at least an hour before bed. The blue light emitted by screens can interfere with the production of **melatonin**, a hormone that regulates sleep.
- Use "night mode" settings or blue light filters if you must use devices in the evening.

8. Get Exposure to Natural Light

- Spend time outdoors during the day to help regulate your circadian rhythm. Morning sunlight, in particular, signals your body when to feel alert and when to wind down.

Music is a universal language that transcends cultural and personal boundaries, resonating with the deepest parts of the human psyche. Music therapy harnesses the power of sound to promote emotional healing and reduce anxiety. This evidence-based therapeutic approach uses music as a tool for expression, relaxation, and connection, offering a safe and creative way to explore and manage emotions.

For individuals struggling with anxiety, music therapy provides an accessible and enjoyable way to calm the mind, regulate emotions, and create a sense of peace. Whether actively engaging with music through playing instruments or passively listening, the benefits of this practice are profound and multifaceted.

The Science Behind Music Therapy

1. Music's Effect on the Brain

Music stimulates multiple areas of the brain, including those involved in emotion, memory, and motor function. It activates the amygdala (emotion regulation), the prefrontal cortex (decision-making), and the hippocampus (memory and learning). This widespread activation explains why music can evoke powerful emotional responses and help regulate mood.

2. The Relaxation Response

Listening to calming music can activate the parasympathetic nervous system, which helps counteract the body's stress response. This results in slower heart rate, lower blood pressure, and reduced levels of cortisol, the stress hormone.

3. Release of Feel-Good Chemicals

Music triggers the release of neurotransmitters like dopamine and serotonin, promoting feelings of joy and relaxation. It also increases the production of oxytocin, a hormone associated with bonding and trust, which can help alleviate feelings of isolation often associated with anxiety.

Music Therapy can be tailored to individual preferences and needs, making it a highly flexible and personalized form of treatment. Common techniques include:

1. Active Participation

- Playing Instruments: Drumming, playing the piano, or using percussion instruments can help channel emotions and release tension.
- Singing: Vocal expression is a powerful way to reduce anxiety and improve breathing patterns.

In guided imagery w/ music, a therapist guides the individual to visualize calming or positive scenarios while listening to soothing music, fostering relaxation and stress reduction.

3. Songwriting

Creating lyrics or composing melodies provides a constructive outlet for expressing emotions that may be difficult to articulate in words.

4. Listening to Music

Carefully curated playlists of calming, uplifting, or personally meaningful songs can evoke positive emotions and alleviate stress.

5. Group Music Therapy

Participating in a choir, band, or drum circle fosters social connection and shared emotional experiences, reducing feelings of isolation.

Benefits of Music Therapy for Anxiety

1. Emotional Regulation: Music therapy helps individuals identify, process, and express emotions in a safe and nonverbal way.
2. Reduction of Physical Symptoms: It can ease physical manifestations of anxiety, such as muscle tension and rapid heart rate.

3. Improved Mood and Relaxation: Music promotes relaxation, reducing feelings of stress and promoting a sense of well-being.
4. Enhanced Focus and Mindfulness: Engaging with music encourages present-moment awareness, interrupting cycles of rumination and worry.
5. Strengthened Social Bonds: Shared musical experiences build connection and community, reducing loneliness and enhancing emotional support.

How to Incorporate Music Therapy into Your Life

While working with a certified music therapist provides the most structured and effective approach, you can also explore music therapy techniques on your own:

1. Create a Personalized Playlist: Compile songs that help you feel calm, joyful, or empowered. Use this playlist during stressful moments or as part of a daily routine.
2. Experiment with Instruments: Even simple instruments like a hand drum, ukulele, or keyboard can provide a creative and soothing outlet.
3. Join a Music Group: Community choirs, drumming circles, or jam sessions offer a space for expression and connection.
4. Practice Guided Relaxation: Pair calming music with meditation or visualization exercises for deeper relaxation.

5. Sing or Hum: Singing releases tension and improves breathing, while humming creates soothing vibrations that can help calm the nervous system.

The Harmony of Healing

Music therapy bridges the gap between body and mind, providing a unique and enriching approach to managing anxiety. Whether it's the steady rhythm of a drumbeat, the soothing melody of a favorite song, or the shared experience of group music-making, music offers a powerful way to connect with yourself and others.

By integrating music therapy into your mental health toolkit, you can unlock a world of emotional healing, creative expression, and inner peace. Let music be the companion that helps guide you through anxious moments, one note at a time.

Chapter 9: Building a Support System
The Importance of Building a Support System

Anxiety can often feel isolating, creating a barrier between you and the people around you. However, one of the most effective ways to manage anxiety is by fostering a strong support system. A network of supportive relationships provides a safe space to share your feelings, seek advice, and gain perspective. Whether it's through friends, family, support groups, or professional connections, a robust support system can make the journey toward mental wellness more manageable and empowering.

This chapter explores the importance of building a support system, the types of support available, and actionable steps to cultivate meaningful connections.

Why a Support System Matters

1. Emotional Support

Having someone to confide in during stressful times can provide relief and validation. Talking about your feelings with a trusted person can help reduce anxiety and prevent you from bottling up emotions.

2. Perspective and Advice

Loved ones and peers can offer fresh perspectives, helping you see situations from a different angle. This can be invaluable when anxiety clouds your judgment or amplifies negative thinking.

3. Encouragement and Motivation

Supportive relationships encourage you to stay on track with treatment plans, self-care routines, and personal goals. Positive reinforcement from others can boost your confidence and resilience.

4. A Sense of Belonging

Knowing you're not alone in your struggles fosters a sense of belonging and reduces feelings of isolation, which are common in those with anxiety.

5. Practical Help

In moments of high stress or crisis, practical support—such as help with errands, childcare, or attending appointments—can alleviate anxiety by lightening your load.

Types of Support Systems

1. Family and Friends

Your closest relationships often form the foundation of your support system. These are the people who know you best and can offer unconditional love and understanding.

2. Support Groups

Joining a support group, either in person or online, connects you with others who have similar experiences. Sharing and listening in such settings can normalize your feelings and provide valuable coping strategies.

3. Mental Health Professionals

Therapists, counselors, and psychiatrists are trained to provide professional guidance tailored to your needs. Regular sessions with a mental health professional can help you navigate complex emotions and develop personalized coping strategies.

4. Community and Social Networks

Faith communities, volunteer organizations, and hobby groups can provide a sense of purpose and belonging, while also expanding your social circle.

5. Workplace Support

Colleagues, mentors, and employee assistance programs can be vital sources of support, especially if work-related stress contributes to your anxiety.

Steps to Build and Strengthen a Support System

1. Identify Your Needs
   - Reflect on the type of support you need most—emotional, practical, or informational.

- Consider the areas in your life where you feel unsupported and who might help fill those gaps.

2. Reach Out

    - Open up to people you trust about your struggles with anxiety. Authenticity often strengthens relationships and invites reciprocal sharing.
    - Don't hesitate to initiate contact. A simple message or call can rekindle connections and show others that you value their presence in your life.

3. Set Boundaries

    - While support is vital, ensure your relationships are balanced and respectful of your boundaries.
    - Avoid overly dependent or toxic relationships that may worsen your anxiety.

4. Join a Group or Community

    - Seek out local or online groups focused on mental health, hobbies, or interests you enjoy. These settings can introduce you to people with shared values or experiences.

5. Practice Gratitude

    - Acknowledge and express appreciation for the support you receive. Gratitude strengthens bonds and fosters a positive feedback loop in relationships.

6. Seek Professional Guidance

- If building or maintaining relationships feels overwhelming, a therapist can provide strategies for improving communication and navigating social interactions.

Overcoming Barriers to Connection

Building a support system can be challenging, especially for those with anxiety. Fear of judgment, feelings of inadequacy, or past negative experiences may hinder your ability to reach out. Here are ways to overcome these barriers:

1. Challenge Negative Thoughts: Reframe fears of rejection or judgment with realistic thinking. For example, "Sharing my feelings may bring me closer to others" is a healthier mindset than "They'll think I'm weak."
2. Start Small: Begin with one trusted person and gradually expand your network.
3. Practice Vulnerability: Being honest about your emotions fosters deeper, more meaningful connections.
4. Be Patient: Building strong relationships takes time. Focus on quality rather than quantity.

The Role of Reciprocity in Support Systems

Healthy support systems thrive on mutual care and respect. While it's important to receive support, offering support to others can also be incredibly fulfilling. Listening to and helping someone else can shift your focus outward, reduce anxiety, and strengthen your relationships.

The Power of Connection

Human beings are inherently social creatures, and a strong support system can be a lifeline during challenging times. The connections you nurture not only provide comfort and guidance but also remind you of your strength and capacity for resilience. By actively building and maintaining a support system, you'll find that anxiety becomes less isolating and more manageable.

Remember, asking for help is not a sign of weakness but an act of courage and self-care. Reach out, connect, and let others walk alongside you on your journey to mental wellness.

The Importance of Communication in Building a Support System

Communication is at the heart of any successful relationship, especially when it comes to managing anxiety. Being able to effectively express your thoughts, feelings, and needs is crucial not only for self-understanding but also for maintaining strong and supportive connections with others. Good communication fosters trust, empathy, and mutual support—key ingredients in a healthy support system.

This section will explore why communication is so essential, how to improve it, and the ways it can strengthen your network of support during difficult times.

Why Communication Matters

1. Clarity of Needs and Boundaries

Clear communication helps others understand what you need and expect from them. Whether it's asking for help with specific tasks, needing someone to listen without offering advice, or setting emotional boundaries, being transparent helps prevent misunderstandings and ensures your needs are met.

2. Strengthening Relationships

When you express yourself honestly and openly, it builds trust in your relationships. Others feel more comfortable opening up as well, creating a deeper bond and mutual respect. Vulnerability and honesty in communication foster a sense of connection, making it easier to receive and give support.

3. Reducing Misunderstandings

Anxiety can sometimes distort how we perceive interactions with others. If you struggle with interpreting body language or reading between the lines, direct communication can clear up any confusion, reducing unnecessary stress or anxiety about social situations.

4. Sharing Your Journey

When you communicate openly about your experiences with anxiety, it normalizes the conversation and helps others understand what you're going through. This is especially important for educating loved ones, friends, or colleagues about how they can support you.

5. Emotional Expression

Being able to express your emotions without fear of judgment is an important part of mental health. Regular, open communication with trusted individuals can provide emotional relief and allow you to process difficult emotions more effectively.

How to Improve Communication in Your Support System

1. Be Honest and Direct

- Express your feelings and needs as clearly as possible. Instead of saying, "I'm feeling off," try, "I'm feeling very anxious today, and I could really use some support."
- Avoid assuming that others can read between the lines. Be upfront about what you need, whether it's emotional support, space, or help with something specific.

2. Use "I" Statements

- Focus on your own feelings and experiences instead of blaming or criticizing others. For example, instead of saying, "You never listen to me," try, "I feel unheard when I share my concerns." This reduces defensiveness and encourages more open dialogue.

3. Listen Actively

- Communication is a two-way street. When someone in your support system shares their thoughts or feelings, practice active listening. This means giving them your full attention, showing empathy, and reflecting back what you've heard. Active listening builds trust and lets others know they are valued.

4. Be Open to Feedback

- Effective communication also involves being open to feedback. If a loved one or therapist offers constructive criticism or suggests ways to manage your anxiety, try to approach the conversation with openness and curiosity. This creates a space for growth and learning.

5. Practice Patience

- Sometimes it may take time for others to understand what you're experiencing or how to best support you. Practice patience as you educate and explain your anxiety to those around you, and don't be discouraged if they don't immediately respond in the way you expect.

While communication is essential for building a supportive network, there are common barriers that can make it difficult to express yourself clearly, including:

1. Fear of Judgment

- The fear of being misunderstood or judged can prevent you from opening up about your struggles. This can be particularly difficult if you're dealing with anxiety and feel that others might not understand. Remember, those who care about you will want to help, not judge you.

2. Emotional Overwhelm

- When anxiety is at its peak, it can be challenging to organize your thoughts or articulate your emotions. In these moments, it can be helpful to write down your feelings before engaging in a conversation, or to simply let the person know that you're struggling to communicate at the moment.

3. Fear of Burdening Others

- You may hesitate to reach out because you don't want to overwhelm others with your problems. However, sharing your feelings and experiences with trusted individuals strengthens the relationship, and most people would rather know what you're going through so they can support you.

- Anxiety can cause you to misinterpret others' body language or tone of voice, which can lead to unnecessary stress. Practicing clear verbal communication, rather than relying solely on non-verbal cues, can help reduce confusion.

Tips for Overcoming Communication Barriers

1. **Be Transparent About Your Struggles**: Let others know that communicating during anxious moments can be difficult for you. This sets realistic expectations and creates understanding.
2. **Practice Self-Compassion**: It's normal to feel nervous about opening up, but be kind to yourself during these times. Even when communication feels difficult, know that each attempt is a step forward.
3. **Use Written Communication**: If verbal communication is too challenging, consider writing down your thoughts and sharing them with a loved one, therapist, or support group. Writing can sometimes feel less intimidating and help organize your emotions.
4. **Seek Professional Help**: A therapist can guide you through communication techniques, especially if anxiety impacts your ability to express yourself clearly. They can also help you navigate sensitive conversations with loved ones.

Building a Support System with Effective Communication

A strong support system is built on mutual trust, respect, and open communication. By expressing yourself honestly, listening actively, and being open to feedback, you create a safe environment where anxiety is understood and supported. Effective communication not only strengthens your relationships but also promotes a sense of connection and belonging, which can reduce feelings of isolation.

Remember, you are not alone in your journey. Whether you're reaching out for comfort, advice, or just a listening ear, effective communication can help you connect with those who are ready to walk alongside you in your mental health journey.

Finding Support Groups: Connecting with Others Who Understand

Support groups offer a powerful opportunity to connect with others who are experiencing similar challenges. For those dealing with anxiety, joining a support group can help normalize your feelings, reduce isolation, and provide valuable insights into coping strategies. Support groups offer a sense of community, allowing you to share experiences, gain empathy, and find strength in numbers.

In this section, we will explore the benefits of support groups, how to find the right one for your needs, and what to expect when participating in a group setting.

The Benefits of Support Groups

1. Shared Experiences and Validation

One of the most powerful aspects of support groups is the opportunity to connect with others who truly understand what you're going through. Hearing similar stories and challenges can be validating and provide reassurance that you're not alone in your struggles.

2. Emotional Support and Empathy

Support groups foster a sense of camaraderie, providing emotional support in a non-judgmental environment. You can share your worries, fears, and triumphs with others who can empathize with your experience, helping to ease feelings of loneliness and isolation.

3. Gaining New Perspectives

Listening to others' experiences can broaden your understanding of anxiety and introduce new coping strategies you may not have considered. Sometimes, the perspectives of fellow group members can offer insights that professional help might not.

4. Accountability and Encouragement

Regular group meetings provide a source of motivation and accountability. When you share your progress and challenges, the group can offer support and encouragement, helping you stay committed to your mental health goals.

5. Reducing Stigma

By participating in a support group, you contribute to breaking down the stigma surrounding anxiety and mental health. These groups offer a space where it's okay to be open and vulnerable about your mental health, making it easier to talk about these topics with others outside the group.

How to Find a Support Group

1. Online Support Groups

In today's digital world, many online communities are dedicated to supporting people with anxiety. Online support groups offer the convenience of connecting from the comfort of your own home. Websites like **Psych Central**, **Anxiety and Depression Association of America (ADAA)**, and social media platforms like **Facebook** or **Reddit** host groups where people with anxiety can share experiences, offer advice, and support one another.

Online groups can be particularly helpful if you live in a rural area or have limited access to in-person meetings. They also allow for flexibility in terms of meeting times and the ability to join groups specific to your type of anxiety or personal interests.

2. In-Person Support Groups

Local support groups often meet at community centers, mental health organizations, hospitals, or private practices. You can search for support groups in your area through:

- **Local mental health organizations**
- **Therapists or counselors**: Many mental health professionals can refer you to reputable in-person groups.
- **Local hospitals or health clinics**: Hospitals often run support groups for mental health or anxiety-related conditions.
- **Social Media Platforms**: Platforms that connect people with similar interests, including mental health and anxiety support groups.

In-person support groups can provide a sense of connection and belonging that may be harder to achieve in online communities. For some, meeting face-to-face helps build trust and provides a deeper level of emotional support.

3. Therapist-Run Support Groups

Many therapists offer group therapy sessions, where individuals with similar concerns—such as anxiety—meet together in a therapeutic setting. These groups often provide a more structured environment, with a licensed professional guiding the discussions and offering therapeutic insights.

You can ask your therapist if they run or can refer you to any group therapy options, or if they can recommend other professional-led groups in your area.

4. Peer-Support Networks

Some organizations, like **The National Alliance on Mental Illness (NAMI)**, run peer-support programs, where individuals with anxiety connect with others who have experienced similar struggles. These peer-support groups are often led by individuals who have lived through mental health challenges, providing a unique understanding of what you're going through.

What to Expect in a Support Group

1. Safe and Confidential Space

Support groups are built on principles of confidentiality and mutual respect. The people you meet in these groups are often there for the same reasons you are, and there is a shared commitment to creating a safe environment where personal experiences and feelings can be shared without judgment.

2. Sharing and Listening

Group meetings often begin with a check-in or roundtable where members can share their current struggles, successes, or questions. You can speak as much or as little as you feel comfortable with, and active listening is encouraged.

3. Emotional Vulnerability

Although it can be intimidating, support groups often require emotional vulnerability. It may be uncomfortable at first, but sharing your experiences and hearing others' stories can help you feel less isolated and more connected.

4. Structured or Unstructured Discussions

Some groups may follow a specific format, such as guided discussions, activities, or readings, while others may be more informal, allowing members to share freely. The format will depend on the group's structure, whether it's peer-led or facilitated by a mental health professional.

5. Encouragement and Support

Throughout the group meeting, members offer support to each other, share helpful tips, and celebrate wins—whether big or small. These moments of encouragement can be empowering and motivate you to keep moving forward in your journey toward healing.

How to choose the right support group. Do you want a group that focuses specifically on anxiety, or are you open to a broader mental health group? Do you prefer in-person meetings, or would online support work better for you?

2. Assess the Group's Structure

Make sure the group's format aligns with your goals. Do you want a more therapeutic environment with a professional facilitator, or are you looking for a casual group where everyone shares freely?

3. Ask About Group Dynamics

Inquire about the size of the group, how long meetings last, and how often they meet. Some people may prefer smaller groups for more intimate discussion, while others might feel more comfortable in larger groups.

4. Trust Your Instincts

When you attend a support group for the first time, trust your gut. If the group feels supportive, inclusive, and safe, it may be a good fit for you. If the environment feels uncomfortable or not aligned with your needs, it's okay to look for another group.

Finding the right support group can be a transformative experience for managing anxiety. Whether it's through shared understanding, practical advice, or emotional support, these communities offer invaluable connections. By joining a group that aligns with your needs and values, you're investing in your mental well-being and building a network of individuals who can provide support, encouragement, and validation.

Don't hesitate to seek out a support group—whether online or in person—because reaching out and connecting with others is a powerful step toward healing and managing anxiety in a healthier, more resilient way.

Involving Family and Friends in Your Journey: Building a Strong Support System

Having the support of family and friends is essential in managing anxiety. While professional help and therapy can provide effective tools for coping, the understanding and emotional support of loved ones can create a network of comfort and encouragement that helps alleviate feelings of isolation and fear. Involving family and friends in your anxiety management journey can provide both practical support and emotional connection, making your path to healing feel less daunting.

Anxiety thrives in isolation, and having family and friends who understand and are empathetic to your needs creates a nurturing environment where you can express your struggles openly. This support system acts as a buffer against stress, offering comfort and reassurance during difficult moments.

1. Reducing Feelings of Stigma

For many, anxiety can feel stigmatizing. You may worry about being judged or misunderstood. Having family and friends who are open to learning about anxiety helps to break down this stigma. It fosters a sense of acceptance and reduces the shame or guilt that can often accompany mental health challenges.

2. Providing Practical Help

Family and friends can offer practical help when you are feeling overwhelmed by anxiety. They can assist with daily tasks, help you stick to routines, and encourage healthy habits like exercise and self-care. They can also offer transportation to appointments, help you prepare for challenging situations, or act as a calming presence during anxiety-provoking moments.

Support from loved ones boosts your self-esteem, reminding you that you are worthy of love, care, and attention despite your struggles. Feeling valued and supported can help reduce negative thoughts about yourself and increase your confidence in managing anxiety.

How to Involve Family and Friends in Your Journey

1. Educate Them About Anxiety

It's important to educate your family and friends about what anxiety is and how it affects you. Many people may not understand that anxiety is a medical condition and not a personal weakness. Explaining the physical and emotional symptoms of anxiety can help your loved ones recognize when you're struggling and understand the challenges you face.

- **Share Resources**: Provide articles, books, or videos that explain anxiety in a way that's easy to understand.
- **Describe Your Experience**: Share how anxiety manifests in your life—whether it's through physical symptoms like a racing heart or through thoughts that spiral out of control. This will help loved ones recognize your triggers and provide the right kind of support.
- **Discuss Coping Strategies**: Let them know what coping strategies work for you (e.g., deep breathing, exercise, or calming techniques) so they can encourage or even help you implement them.

2. Set Clear Expectations and Boundaries

Communicating your needs clearly is essential. Family and friends may want to help, but they may not always know how. Setting boundaries is crucial in ensuring that your relationships remain healthy and supportive.

- **Be Honest About Your Limits**: If you need time alone to recharge, let your loved ones know. If you need them to listen without offering solutions, communicate that too.
- **Ask for Specific Help**: Be direct about the type of support you need. For instance, you might need them to help you stay grounded during a panic attack or just to provide a distraction when you feel overwhelmed.
- **Respect Their Boundaries**: While it's important to have support, it's also crucial to respect the boundaries of your loved ones. Don't be afraid to discuss how much support feels comfortable for both you and them.

3. Involve Them in Therapy (When Appropriate)

In some cases, family therapy or involving loved ones in therapy sessions can help them better understand your anxiety. Many therapists offer family therapy as a way to educate family members, improve communication, and help everyone develop better coping strategies.

- **Attend Sessions Together**: If you're comfortable, ask your therapist if they would be willing to include your loved ones in a session or two to discuss ways they can be supportive.

- **Communication Tools**: Learn effective communication strategies together so that you can express your needs and feelings more clearly.

4. Encourage Open Communication

Building a relationship of open communication with your family and friends is vital. Let them know when you are feeling anxious and what they can do to support you. Keep the lines of communication open, even when you're not feeling anxious. Regularly checking in with each other can prevent misunderstandings and strengthen the bond between you.

- **Share Your Progress**: Talk about what strategies are working and what challenges you're facing. This helps your family and friends stay involved in your healing journey.
- **Express Appreciation**: Acknowledge their efforts and thank them for their support. This reinforces their willingness to continue helping you in meaningful ways.

5. Encourage Self-Care for Your Loved Ones

Caring for someone with anxiety can be challenging, and it's important for your family and friends to take care of themselves as well. Encourage them to practice self-care, seek support if needed, and take breaks when necessary.

Sometimes, despite your best efforts, family and friends may resist supporting you in the way that you need. They may not understand the severity of your anxiety, or they might be reluctant to change their approach to helping. Here are some ways to manage resistance:

1. Stay Patient and Persistent

Changing someone's perspective takes time. Be patient and persistent in your efforts to communicate your needs. Share resources and examples of how their support can make a difference in your anxiety management.

2. Seek Outside Help

If resistance persists and becomes a barrier to your progress, consider seeking help from a therapist who can help mediate conversations or offer guidance on how to educate and involve your loved ones.

3. Find Other Sources of Support

If family or friends are not able to offer the support you need, remember that you can turn to other sources—such as support groups, a therapist, or online communities—where you can receive the empathy and care that you deserve.

Creating a Supportive Environment at Home

A supportive home environment plays a huge role in managing anxiety. Here are some ways to foster this kind of environment:

1. Create a Calm Space

Establish a physical space at home where you can retreat when feeling overwhelmed. This could be a quiet corner, a cozy chair, or even a bedroom. Fill this space with calming elements, such as soft lighting, plants, or soothing sounds, to help reduce anxiety.

2. Foster Healthy Routines

Anxiety thrives on unpredictability. Having a regular routine at home—especially regarding sleep, meals, and self-care—can provide stability and help reduce feelings of chaos. Family and friends can support you in maintaining these routines by encouraging healthy habits, such as eating balanced meals or taking regular breaks.

3. Encourage Positive Interactions

Foster an environment of positivity by encouraging supportive and reassuring words. Avoid criticism or dismissing your anxiety, as this can make you feel invalidated. Instead, focus on listening, understanding, and offering gentle encouragement.

Involving family and friends in your journey with anxiety can be a transformative experience. When done thoughtfully and with clear communication, the support of your loved ones can make managing anxiety feel more manageable. By educating them, setting boundaries, and encouraging empathy and understanding, you create a support network that not only helps you cope with anxiety but also strengthens the bonds you share.

Remember, while family and friends can provide important emotional and practical support, you are the expert in your own journey. It's crucial to advocate for yourself, communicate openly, and seek professional help when necessary. Together with your loved ones, you can navigate the challenges of anxiety and move toward greater mental well-being.

Having the support of family and friends is essential in managing anxiety. While professional help and therapy can provide effective tools for coping, the understanding and emotional support of loved ones can create a network of comfort and encouragement that helps alleviate feelings of isolation and fear. Involving family and friends in your anxiety management journey can provide both practical support and emotional connection, making your path to healing feel less daunting.

This section will explore how to involve your loved ones in your mental health journey, how to educate them about anxiety, and how to establish a supportive environment at home.

Why Involving Family and Friends is Important

1. Creating a Supportive Environment

Anxiety thrives in isolation, and having family and friends who understand and are empathetic to your needs creates a nurturing environment where you can express your struggles openly. This support system acts as a buffer against stress, offering comfort and reassurance during difficult moments.

2. Reducing Feelings of Stigma

For many, anxiety can feel stigmatizing. You may worry about being judged or misunderstood. Having family and friends who are open to learning about anxiety helps to break down this stigma. It fosters a sense of acceptance and reduces the shame or guilt that can often accompany mental health challenges.

3. Providing Practical Help

Family and friends can offer practical help when you are feeling overwhelmed by anxiety. They can assist with daily tasks, help you stick to routines, and encourage healthy habits like exercise and self-care. They can also offer transportation to appointments, help you prepare for challenging situations, or act as a calming presence during anxiety-provoking moments.

4. Boosting Self-Esteem and Confidence

Support from loved ones boosts your self-esteem, reminding you that you are worthy of love, care, and attention despite your struggles. Feeling valued and supported can help reduce negative thoughts about yourself and increase your confidence in managing anxiety.

How to Involve Family and Friends in Your Journey

1. Educate Them About Anxiety

It's important to educate your family and friends about what anxiety is and how it affects you. Many people may not understand that anxiety is a medical condition and not a personal weakness. Explaining the physical and emotional symptoms of anxiety can help your loved ones recognize when you're struggling and understand the challenges you face.

- **Share Resources**: Provide articles, books, or videos that explain anxiety in a way that's easy to understand.
- **Describe Your Experience**: Share how anxiety manifests in your life—whether it's through physical symptoms like a racing heart or through thoughts that spiral out of control. This will help loved ones recognize your triggers and provide the right kind of support.
- **Discuss Coping Strategies**: Let them know what coping strategies work for you (e.g., deep breathing, exercise, or calming techniques) so they can encourage or even help you implement them.

2. Set Clear Expectations and Boundaries

Communicating your needs clearly is essential. Family and friends may want to help, but they may not always know how. Setting boundaries is crucial in ensuring that your relationships remain healthy and supportive.

- **Be Honest About Your Limits**: If you need time alone to recharge, let your loved ones know. If you need them to listen without offering solutions, communicate that too.
- **Ask for Specific Help**: Be direct about the type of support you need. For instance, you might need them to help you stay grounded during a panic attack or just to provide a distraction when you feel overwhelmed.
- **Respect Their Boundaries**: While it's important to have support, it's also crucial to respect the boundaries of your loved ones. Don't be afraid to discuss how much support feels comfortable for both you and them.

3. Involve Them in Therapy (When Appropriate)

In some cases, family therapy or involving loved ones in therapy sessions can help them better understand your anxiety. Many therapists offer family therapy as a way to educate family members, improve communication, and help everyone develop better coping strategies.

- **Attend Sessions Together**: If you're comfortable, ask your therapist if they would be willing to include your loved ones in a session or two to discuss ways they can be supportive.

- **Communication Tools**: Learn effective communication strategies together so that you can express your needs and feelings more clearly.

4. Encourage Open Communication

Building a relationship of open communication with your family and friends is vital. Let them know when you are feeling anxious and what they can do to support you. Keep the lines of communication open, even when you're not feeling anxious. Regularly checking in with each other can prevent misunderstandings and strengthen the bond between you.

- **Share Your Progress**: Talk about what strategies are working and what challenges you're facing. This helps your family and friends stay involved in your healing journey.
- **Express Appreciation**: Acknowledge their efforts and thank them for their support. This reinforces their willingness to continue helping you in meaningful ways.

5. Encourage Self-Care for Your Loved Ones

Caring for someone with anxiety can be challenging, and it's important for your family and friends to take care of themselves as well. Encourage them to practice self-care, seek support if needed, and take breaks when necessary. The more balanced and healthy they feel, the better able they will be to support you effectively.

What to Do if You Encounter Resistance

Sometimes, despite your best efforts, family and friends may resist supporting you in the way that you need. They may not understand the severity of your anxiety, or they might be reluctant to change their approach to helping. Here are some ways to manage resistance:

1. Stay Patient and Persistent

Changing someone's perspective takes time. Be patient and persistent in your efforts to communicate your needs. Share resources and examples of how their support can make a difference in your anxiety management.

2. Seek Outside Help

If resistance persists and becomes a barrier to your progress, consider seeking help from a therapist who can help mediate conversations or offer guidance on how to educate and involve your loved ones.

3. Find Other Sources of Support

If family or friends are not able to offer the support you need, remember that you can turn to other sources—such as support groups, a therapist, or online communities—where you can receive the empathy and care that you deserve.

Creating a Supportive Environment at Home

A supportive home environment plays a huge role in managing anxiety. Here are some ways to foster this kind of environment:

1. Create a Calm Space

Establish a physical space at home where you can retreat when feeling overwhelmed. This could be a quiet corner, a cozy chair, or even a bedroom. Fill this space with calming elements, such as soft lighting, plants, or soothing sounds, to help reduce anxiety.

2. Foster Healthy Routines

Anxiety thrives on unpredictability. Having a regular routine at home—especially regarding sleep, meals, and self-care—can provide stability and help reduce feelings of chaos. Family and friends can support you in maintaining these routines by encouraging healthy habits, such as eating balanced meals or taking regular breaks.

3. Encourage Positive Interactions

Foster an environment of positivity by encouraging supportive and reassuring words. Avoid criticism or dismissing your anxiety, as this can make you feel invalidated. Instead, focus on listening, understanding, and offering gentle encouragement.

Empowering Your Support System

Involving family and friends in your journey with anxiety can be a transformative experience. When done thoughtfully and with clear communication, the support of your loved ones can make managing anxiety feel more manageable. By educating them, setting boundaries, and encouraging empathy and understanding, you create a support network that not only helps you cope with anxiety but also strengthens the bonds you share.

Remember, while family and friends can provide important emotional and practical support, you are the expert in your own journey. It's crucial to advocate for yourself, communicate openly, and seek professional help when necessary. Together with your loved ones, you can navigate the challenges of anxiety and move toward greater mental well-being.

Animal-Assisted Therapy: Finding Comfort and Connection in Four-Legged Companions

Animal-assisted therapy (AAT) is a therapeutic approach that involves the use of animals, typically dogs or horses, to help individuals manage emotional and psychological challenges.

For people suffering from anxiety, animal-assisted therapy offers unique benefits that can provide both immediate relief and long-term support. The bond between humans and animals can help reduce anxiety, provide emotional comfort, and encourage mindfulness, making it easier for individuals to shift their focus away from their own worries and self-criticism.

This section will explore how animal-assisted therapy works, the benefits it offers for anxiety, and how it helps anxious individuals break free from their own thoughts by focusing on the well-being of the animal, fostering a sense of connection, and providing opportunities for healing.

How Animal-Assisted Therapy Helps Alleviate Anxiety

1. Promoting Emotional Regulation

Animals can act as a grounding presence, offering emotional support when anxiety overwhelms the individual. Their non-judgmental and unconditional love creates a safe space where anxious individuals can feel comforted without fear of criticism or rejection. Petting or spending time with an animal has been shown to lower stress hormone levels (like cortisol) and increase levels of oxytocin, a hormone associated with bonding and relaxation.

The simple act of petting an animal can calm the nervous system, allowing individuals to feel less tense and more connected to the present moment, which reduces the overwhelming feelings of anxiety. This physical interaction can also distract from anxious thoughts and provide a sense of calm.

2. Encouraging Mindfulness and Present-Moment Awareness

Anxiety often arises from dwelling on past regrets or fearing future events. Animal-assisted therapy helps individuals focus on the present by directing their attention to the animal's needs, behaviors, and emotions. For example, while interacting with a therapy animal, the person might focus on the animal's well-being, needs (such as feeding, grooming, or playing), and body language, effectively drawing attention away from their anxious thoughts.

Mindfulness is a core aspect of managing anxiety, and animal-assisted therapy encourages this through the need for direct, present-moment engagement with the animal. Focusing on the animal's needs—whether it's a gentle touch, a soothing voice, or playful interaction—redirects the individual's attention and helps them become more aware of the moment rather than the anxiety-producing thoughts in their mind.

3. Building Emotional Connection

Animals, especially dogs and horses, are known for their ability to connect emotionally with humans. Many animals have an innate sense of empathy and can respond to their owner's emotional state, often offering comfort when needed most. For people with anxiety, this can create a profound sense of companionship and emotional safety.

The act of bonding with an animal can evoke feelings of trust, joy, and unconditional love. This bond can counteract feelings of isolation and loneliness that often accompany anxiety. For some individuals, an animal can become a non-judgmental "companion" who provides a sense of stability, helping the individual feel grounded and supported.

Breaking the Cycle of Self-Focus: Thinking About Others Through Animal-Assisted Therapy

For those suffering from anxiety, the constant cycle of negative self-talk and worry can often lead to a distorted sense of reality. The mind becomes fixated on what might go wrong, on personal shortcomings, or on the fear of impending catastrophe. This "headspace" often limits one's ability to focus on anything outside of themselves, leading to heightened anxiety and a sense of helplessness.

Animal-assisted therapy offers a natural, effective way to shift the focus away from one's own worries by encouraging the individual to care for and nurture another being.

1. Fostering Compassion and Empathy

Animals have an amazing way of drawing out compassion and empathy. As the individual becomes more attuned to the animal's needs—whether it's feeding, walking, or simply sitting with them—they begin to focus less on their internal fears and more on the well-being of the animal. This shift in focus can help break the self-referential cycle that often drives anxiety.

In addition, caring for an animal can help develop a sense of responsibility and purpose. Taking care of an animal provides an opportunity to give love and attention without worrying about how the animal might feel about them. This helps the individual step outside their own internal thoughts and gain perspective on the relationship, which can lead to feelings of self-worth and accomplishment.

2. Offering a Sense of Purpose

For individuals with anxiety, daily life can sometimes feel overwhelming, with constant rumination and overthinking. Caring for an animal can provide a structured, purposeful activity, offering a healthy distraction and motivating individuals to engage in life outside of their own headspace. Routine tasks like feeding, walking, or playing with an animal help to create a sense of normalcy and accomplishment, counteracting the feeling of being overwhelmed by internal struggles.

Anxiety can sometimes feel like a never-ending loop of worry, but when a person shifts their attention to something tangible, like the needs of a therapy animal, they break free from the paralysis that anxiety can cause. By focusing on an external task, they can experience the satisfaction of nurturing and caring for another being, which fosters a sense of purpose and accomplishment.

3. Enhancing Social Interaction

While anxiety often leads to social withdrawal, therapy animals, especially dogs, can provide a bridge for social interaction. Therapy animals often serve as social catalysts, encouraging their owners to engage with others in a safe and non-threatening way. For example, walking a dog in the park may naturally lead to conversations with other dog owners or even passersby, allowing individuals with anxiety to practice social skills in a low-pressure environment.

Animals are also an excellent conversation starter and can help ease the tension in social situations. Having a pet as a companion reduces the pressure to perform socially and instead provides an opportunity for the individual to focus on the animal's needs and behavior.

Benefits of Animal-Assisted Therapy for Different Types of Anxiety

1. Generalized Anxiety Disorder (GAD)

For those with generalized anxiety, constant worrying can feel like an exhausting and unrelenting cycle. Animal-assisted therapy can help disrupt this cycle by offering moments of calm, grounding the person in the present, and providing a natural distraction from anxious thoughts. The bond formed with a therapy animal encourages positive engagement, reducing the focus on future fears and promoting a healthier emotional balance.

2. Social Anxiety

Social anxiety often leads to avoidance of social interactions due to fears of judgment or rejection. Having a therapy animal can make socializing easier, as the individual feels less self-conscious and more at ease. The presence of the animal provides a source of comfort and security, making social situations feel less threatening. Therapy animals can also encourage the development of healthy social behaviors, such as initiating conversation or engaging with others in a relaxed setting.

3. Panic Disorder

Panic attacks can feel overwhelming, with intense physical symptoms such as rapid heartbeat, shortness of breath, and dizziness. During a panic attack, animal-assisted therapy can help provide immediate comfort. The presence of an animal, particularly a trained therapy dog, can provide emotional support by offering a calming influence and helping the individual stay grounded. The act of focusing on the animal's behavior or presence can shift attention away from the physical sensations of panic and help bring the person back to a state of calm.

The Healing Power of Animals

Animal-assisted therapy is a unique and effective way to help individuals with anxiety move out of their own heads and focus on the needs of their animal companions. By providing emotional support, grounding techniques, and opportunities for connection, therapy animals offer a sense of comfort and relief during moments of stress. The bond between humans and animals not only helps reduce anxiety symptoms but also promotes mindfulness, empathy, and compassion.

For many, the companionship of a therapy animal provides a vital lifeline, offering both immediate comfort and long-term healing benefits. Through animal-assisted therapy, individuals with anxiety can find solace in the unconditional love of their furry companions, creating a healthier, more balanced life with reduced anxiety and greater emotional resilience.

Chapter 10: When to Seek Professional Help

When to Seek Professional Help

Managing anxiety is a journey that can often be navigated with self-care strategies, lifestyle changes, and support from loved ones. However, there are times when anxiety can become overwhelming and difficult to manage on your own. Recognizing when professional help is necessary is an essential step in managing anxiety and ensuring that you have the resources and support you need to cope effectively.

This chapter will explore the signs that indicate it might be time to seek professional help for anxiety, the types of mental health professionals who can assist, and what to expect when you reach out for support.

When to Recognize That Anxiety Requires Professional Help

While feeling anxious from time to time is a normal part of life, excessive or chronic anxiety can significantly impact your well-being and ability to function. It's important to recognize the warning signs that your anxiety may be becoming more than you can handle on your own and that professional intervention could be beneficial.

1. Anxiety Interferes with Daily Life

One of the key indicators that it might be time to seek professional help is when anxiety begins to interfere with your daily activities. If your anxious thoughts or physical symptoms are preventing you from going to work, school, or engaging in social activities, it's a clear sign that you may need additional support.

For example, if you're avoiding tasks or isolating yourself due to fear or anxiety, or if your productivity at work or school is declining, it might be time to reach out for help. Anxiety that hinders your ability to maintain relationships or fulfill daily responsibilities is a significant red flag.

2. The Anxiety Is Persistent and Unrelenting

Anxiety is often a response to stress or a specific situation, but when it becomes persistent, chronic, or overwhelming, it can be a sign of a more serious issue. If you find that your anxiety is present for most of the day, every day, and is not linked to any specific stressor, it may be time to speak to a mental health professional.

Symptoms that are present for weeks or months and continue to intensify may indicate the development of a generalized anxiety disorder (GAD) or another anxiety-related condition.

3. Physical Symptoms Are Becoming Unmanageable

Anxiety doesn't just affect the mind—it also manifests physically. If you're experiencing physical symptoms such as chest pain, rapid heartbeat, shortness of breath, dizziness, or gastrointestinal issues (such as nausea or stomach cramps) regularly due to anxiety, it's important to seek professional guidance. These symptoms can be signs of a panic disorder, and in some cases, they may even mimic medical conditions like heart problems.

Persistent physical symptoms that are related to anxiety should not be ignored, especially if they are impacting your health and well-being. A mental health professional can help you understand how anxiety is affecting your body and work with you to develop strategies for managing the physical and emotional symptoms.

4. You Are Struggling with Coping Strategies

Everyone experiences anxiety, but when you find that the strategies you've used to cope with anxiety—whether it's deep breathing, exercise, or talking with friends—are no longer effective, it may be time to seek professional help. Mental health professionals can offer more targeted, evidence-based therapies like cognitive-behavioral therapy (CBT) or mindfulness-based therapies that may be more effective in addressing persistent or severe anxiety.

If your attempts to manage anxiety on your own no longer seem to be working, reaching out to a therapist or counselor can provide you with the tools and coping mechanisms needed to regain control over your life.

5. You're Experiencing Symptoms of Depression

Anxiety and depression are often linked, and it's common for someone with chronic anxiety to also experience depression. If your anxiety is accompanied by feelings of sadness, hopelessness, a lack of interest in things you once enjoyed, or a sense of emotional numbness, it's important to seek professional help immediately.

Depression can make it harder to manage anxiety, and vice versa. A therapist or mental health professional can help address both conditions simultaneously, improving your overall mental health and quality of life.

6. You Have Thoughts of Self-Harm or Suicide

If you find yourself thinking about self-harm, suicide, or having thoughts of harming others, it's critical to seek professional help immediately. These thoughts are serious and require immediate attention from a mental health professional. A therapist, counselor, or psychiatrist can provide support, create a safety plan, and offer therapeutic interventions that can help you manage your emotions and begin the healing process.

It's important to remember that seeking help when experiencing thoughts of self-harm or suicide is a brave and necessary step toward feeling better. Reaching out for support is crucial to your well-being.

Types of Mental Health Professionals Who Can Help

There are various mental health professionals who can help you manage anxiety, and it's important to know who to turn to depending on your needs. Here are some common options:

1. Psychiatrists

Psychiatrists are medical doctors who specialize in diagnosing and treating mental health conditions, including anxiety disorders. They are qualified to prescribe medication, and they can help you determine if medication might be necessary in your treatment plan.

If your anxiety is severe and requires medication or if you have symptoms of other mental health conditions (such as depression), a psychiatrist can provide a comprehensive treatment plan that includes both medication and therapy.

2. Psychologists

Psychologists are trained mental health professionals who specialize in therapy and psychological assessments. They provide talk therapy, including cognitive-behavioral therapy (CBT), which is effective for treating anxiety. Psychologists help individuals understand their thoughts, feelings, and behaviors, and they can teach coping strategies to manage anxiety more effectively.

Psychologists typically do not prescribe medication but work closely with other healthcare professionals to provide holistic care.

3. Licensed Therapists and Counselors

Therapists and counselors are trained to provide various forms of talk therapy, including CBT, dialectical behavior therapy (DBT), mindfulness-based therapy, and other interventions that can help with anxiety. They are licensed professionals who can offer support in managing anxiety through one-on-one or group therapy sessions.

Therapists can be licensed social workers (LCSWs), marriage and family therapists (LMFTs), or professional counselors (LPCs), and they typically specialize in different types of therapy and approaches to mental health care.

4. Psychiatric Nurse Practitioners

Psychiatric nurse practitioners (NPs) are advanced practice nurses with specialized training in mental health care. They can diagnose mental health conditions, prescribe medication, and provide psychotherapy. They often work in conjunction with psychiatrists to create comprehensive treatment plans for patients with anxiety.

Psychiatric nurse practitioners are especially helpful if you need both medication and therapy to manage your anxiety symptoms.

5. Support Groups

While not a substitute for individual therapy, support groups offer a sense of community and shared experience. Joining a support group for anxiety can provide you with a safe space to talk about your struggles, hear from others who are going through similar challenges, and find encouragement. Many support groups are facilitated by trained mental health professionals, but peer-led groups can also be a valuable resource.

Support groups can be an additional form of support when you're feeling isolated or unsure about your anxiety journey.

What to Expect When Seeking Professional Help

The process of seeking professional help for anxiety can feel daunting, but it's an important step in taking control of your mental health. Here's what you can expect when you reach out to a mental health professional:

1. Initial Consultation

Your first meeting with a mental health professional will likely involve an intake or assessment session. During this session, the therapist or psychiatrist will ask about your symptoms, medical history, and any triggers or factors contributing to your anxiety. Be honest and open about what you're experiencing so they can provide the most accurate diagnosis and treatment plan.

2. Diagnosis and Treatment Plan

Based on the information gathered during the assessment, the mental health professional will provide a diagnosis and recommend a treatment plan. Treatment may include therapy (such as CBT, exposure therapy, or mindfulness-based therapies), medication, or a combination of both.

3. Regular Sessions

If therapy is part of your treatment plan, you will attend regular sessions (usually weekly or biweekly) to work on managing your anxiety. During therapy, you will learn coping strategies, work through any unresolved issues, and develop skills to manage stress and anxiety more effectively.

4. Follow-up and Adjustment

Your treatment plan will be adjusted over time as you progress. If you're prescribed medication, regular follow-up appointments with a psychiatrist or nurse practitioner will help monitor its effectiveness and address any side effects. Therapy sessions will evolve as you learn new coping techniques and work through your anxieties.

Conclusion: Taking the First Step

Seeking professional help for anxiety can feel intimidating, but it's an important step in improving your mental health and well-being. If your anxiety is interfering with your daily life, physical health, or relationships, it's crucial to reach out for support. A mental health professional can provide the guidance, strategies, and tools you need to manage anxiety more effectively and lead a fulfilling life.

Remember, there's no shame in asking for help. In fact, it's a courageous and proactive step toward healing. Whether it's through therapy, medication, or a combination of both, the right professional support can make a world of difference in your journey to manage anxiety.

Medication Options for Anxiety Disorders

While therapy and lifestyle changes are key components of managing anxiety, medication can also play a significant role, especially when symptoms are severe or persistent. Medication can help reduce the intensity of anxiety symptoms, making it easier for individuals to engage in therapy, practice coping strategies, and function in daily life. However, medication is typically considered part of a broader treatment plan, which may include therapy, lifestyle changes, and support systems.

In this section, we'll explore the different types of medications commonly used to treat anxiety disorders, their potential benefits, side effects, and considerations when discussing medication options with your healthcare provider.

1. Anti-Anxiety Medications (Anxiolytics)

Anxiolytics are a class of drugs designed to reduce anxiety symptoms. The most commonly prescribed anxiolytics are **benzodiazepines**, which are fast-acting medications that can help calm acute anxiety and panic symptoms. They are usually prescribed for short-term use due to their potential for dependence and tolerance.

Benzodiazepines:

- **Examples:** Diazepam (Valium), Lorazepam (Ativan), Alprazolam (Xanax), Clonazepam (Klonopin)
- **How they work:** Benzodiazepines work by enhancing the effects of a neurotransmitter called **gamma-aminobutyric acid** (GABA), which inhibits activity in the brain, leading to a calming effect on the nervous system. This makes benzodiazepines particularly effective for reducing the acute symptoms of anxiety, such as restlessness, tension, and panic attacks.
- **Pros:**
    - Quick onset of relief (within 30-60 minutes).
    - Effective in treating acute anxiety and panic attacks.
- **Cons:**
    - Risk of dependence and tolerance with long-term use.
    - Potential for withdrawal symptoms if stopped abruptly.
    - Can cause drowsiness, dizziness, or impaired coordination, which may interfere with daily functioning.

While benzodiazepines can offer quick relief for anxiety symptoms, they are generally used on a short-term or as-needed basis due to their potential for misuse and dependence. For long-term management of anxiety disorders, other medications are often preferred.

2. Selective Serotonin Reuptake Inhibitors (SSRIs)

SSRIs are a class of **antidepressants** that are commonly used to treat anxiety disorders. They work by increasing the level of **serotonin**, a neurotransmitter that plays a key role in mood regulation. SSRIs are considered first-line treatment for generalized anxiety disorder (GAD), panic disorder, social anxiety disorder, and other anxiety-related conditions.

Common SSRIs include:

- **Examples:** Sertraline (Zoloft), Fluoxetine (Prozac), Escitalopram (Lexapro), Paroxetine (Paxil), Citalopram (Celexa)
- **How they work:** SSRIs prevent the reabsorption (reuptake) of serotonin in the brain, leading to increased serotonin levels in the synaptic gaps between neurons.

Pros:

- Fewer side effects compared to older antidepressants (e.g., tricyclic antidepressants).
- Not addictive.
- Can help treat both anxiety and depression simultaneously, as they are often comorbid conditions.

Cons:

- Initial side effects can include nausea, sleep disturbances, dizziness, or sexual dysfunction.
- Full therapeutic effects may take 4-6 weeks to be felt.
- Possible side effects may lead to discontinuation or dose adjustments.

Considerations:

SSRIs are typically prescribed for long-term use and may be combined with therapy for best results. While they are generally well-tolerated, it's important to have regular follow-ups with a doctor to monitor for side effects and ensure the medication is working effectively.

Serotonin-Norepinephrine Reuptake Inhibitors (SNRIs) are a class of antidepressants that are used to treat anxiety disorders. Like SSRIs, SNRIs increase serotonin levels, but they also increase the levels of **norepinephrine**, a neurotransmitter involved in the body's stress response.

Common SNRIs include:

- **Examples:** Venlafaxine (Effexor XR), Duloxetine (Cymbalta)
- **How they work:** SNRIs prevent the reuptake of both serotonin and norepinephrine, leading to increased levels of both neurotransmitters in the brain. This can help regulate mood, alleviate anxiety, and reduce physical symptoms of anxiety, such as muscle tension.
- **Pros:**
    - Effective for generalized anxiety disorder, social anxiety, and panic disorder.
    - Can help alleviate both anxiety and depressive symptoms.
    - Less risk of dependence or misuse compared to benzodiazepines.
- **Cons:**
    - Similar to SSRIs, side effects can include nausea, dizziness, and sexual dysfunction.
    - May cause an increase in blood pressure (especially with higher doses), which requires monitoring.
    - Withdrawal symptoms can occur if the medication is stopped abruptly.

SNRIs are effective for long-term anxiety management and can also help with chronic pain conditions like fibromyalgia or neuropathy. As with SSRIs, it's important to work with a healthcare provider to monitor progress and side effects.

4. Beta-Blockers

While beta-blockers are primarily used to treat heart conditions, they are sometimes prescribed for short-term anxiety management, particularly in cases of performance anxiety or situational anxiety (such as before public speaking or a big event). Beta-blockers help control the physical symptoms of anxiety by blocking the effects of adrenaline, which is responsible for symptoms like rapid heart rate and trembling.

Common beta-blockers include:

- **Examples:** Propranolol (Inderal), Atenolol (Tenormin)
- **How they work:** Beta-blockers block the effects of norepinephrine and epinephrine (adrenaline), which helps reduce physical symptoms like a racing heart, shaking, and sweating during anxious moments. While they do not reduce anxious thoughts, they can help calm the body's stress response.
- **Pros:**
    - Effective in controlling physical symptoms of anxiety, especially in performance situations.
    - Generally well-tolerated with few side effects.

- **Cons:**
    - Do not address the emotional or cognitive aspects of anxiety.
    - Not effective for chronic anxiety or panic disorder.
    - Can cause fatigue, dizziness, or cold extremities.

Considerations:

Beta-blockers are generally recommended for specific situations (such as public speaking or before a stressful event), rather than for daily management of anxiety. They can provide effective relief for physical symptoms but are not a long-term solution for ongoing anxiety.

5. Benzodiazepines for Short-Term Relief

Though benzodiazepines are generally not recommended for long-term use due to the risk of dependence, they can still be used for **short-term relief** or for situations where immediate relief is needed, such as during a panic attack. They are typically prescribed in conjunction with other therapies or medications.

Benzodiazepines promote relaxation by enhancing the effects of GABA in the brain. This rapid onset of action can make them effective in treating acute anxiety and panic attacks. However, their sedative properties can lead to dependence if used over time.

Pros:

- Quick relief from acute anxiety symptoms.
- Effective in managing panic attacks and severe anxiety episodes.

Cons:

- High potential for misuse, dependence, and tolerance.
- Side effects such as sedation, dizziness, impaired coordination, and memory problems.
- Typically not recommended for long-term use due to risk of addiction.

Considerations:

Benzodiazepines should only be used under close supervision by a healthcare provider, and typically for short periods or as needed. If you find that you are relying on these medications frequently, it may be time to explore longer-term treatment options.

Medication can play an important role in managing anxiety, particularly when symptoms are severe or persistent. It can help stabilize mood, alleviate physical symptoms, and make it easier for individuals to engage in other therapeutic practices like Cognitive Behavioral Therapy (CBT) and mindfulness techniques.

However, medication is often most effective when used as part of a comprehensive treatment plan, which includes therapy, lifestyle changes, and self-care practices. It is essential to work closely with a healthcare provider to find the medication that best suits your needs and to monitor its effectiveness over time. With the right combination of medication, therapy, and support, managing anxiety becomes more manageable, allowing individuals to regain control over their lives and mental health.

What to Expect in Therapy

When seeking professional help for anxiety, one of the first steps is to engage in therapy. Therapy can be a powerful tool for understanding the root causes of anxiety, learning new coping strategies, and addressing any underlying emotional or psychological issues. However, starting therapy can be intimidating, especially if you're not sure what to expect. Understanding the process can help alleviate some of the uncertainty and set you up for a more successful therapeutic experience.

In this section, we will explore what you can expect when you begin therapy for anxiety, including the different types of therapy, the process of finding the right therapist, and how therapy can help you manage and overcome your anxiety.

1. The Therapeutic Process: Getting Started

The first step in therapy for anxiety typically involves an initial consultation or intake session. During this session, the therapist will gather important information about your background, your anxiety symptoms, and any related issues (such as depression, trauma, or stress). You will likely be asked questions about your emotional state, lifestyle, and how your anxiety affects your daily life. The therapist may also discuss your goals for therapy and explain the therapeutic process.

What to Expect:

- Assessment: Your therapist will ask questions to better understand the nature and severity of your anxiety. They may also ask about any past experiences with therapy or medications.
- Goal Setting: You will have the opportunity to discuss what you hope to achieve in therapy. Whether it's managing panic attacks, reducing general anxiety, or addressing specific triggers, this is an important step in creating a treatment plan.
- Explanation of Therapy Options: Your therapist will likely explain the different approaches to therapy that might be helpful for you, including Cognitive Behavioral Therapy (CBT), mindfulness-based therapy, or other modalities.

The initial session may last anywhere from 45 minutes to an hour, and it's important to know that this is just the beginning of your journey. You will not necessarily feel "cured" after one session, but you will gain insights into the process and feel more comfortable with the idea of therapy.

2. Types of Therapy for Anxiety

There are many different types of therapy that can help with anxiety, and it's important to find an approach that resonates with you. Below are some of the most commonly used therapeutic modalities for treating anxiety:

Cognitive Behavioral Therapy (CBT):

CBT is one of the most widely used and researched therapies for anxiety. It focuses on identifying and changing negative thought patterns that contribute to anxiety. In CBT, you'll work with your therapist to recognize irrational thoughts, challenge them, and replace them with more balanced and realistic beliefs.

- What to Expect: CBT is structured and goal-oriented. You'll work with your therapist to identify specific anxiety-provoking situations and learn strategies to reframe your thinking and reduce the anxiety response.
- Duration: Typically short-term (12-20 sessions), with weekly or bi-weekly appointments.

Exposure Therapy:

Exposure therapy is a subset of CBT that focuses on confronting feared situations in a controlled and gradual way. The goal is to reduce fear over time by desensitizing yourself to triggers in a safe environment.

- What to Expect: Exposure therapy may involve gradual exposure to the anxiety-provoking situation, starting with less stressful scenarios and gradually increasing in difficulty. You may be asked to imagine the situation first, then gradually face it in real life.
- Duration: Can vary depending on the individual's progress, but it typically takes several sessions.

Mindfulness-Based Stress Reduction (MBSR):

MBSR is a therapeutic approach that incorporates mindfulness and meditation practices to help individuals manage stress and anxiety. It emphasizes being present in the moment and observing your thoughts without judgment.

- What to Expect: You will learn meditation techniques and mindfulness exercises that help you become more aware of your thoughts and emotions. You will be encouraged to practice mindfulness outside of therapy to develop a greater sense of awareness and control over your anxiety.
- Duration: MBSR programs typically run for 8 weeks, with weekly sessions and daily practices.

Acceptance and Commitment Therapy (ACT):

ACT focuses on accepting negative thoughts and feelings instead of trying to eliminate them. The therapy teaches individuals to live according to their values and take action even in the presence of anxiety.

- What to Expect: You'll learn techniques to embrace difficult emotions and thoughts without letting them control your behavior. You will also work on setting meaningful life goals that align with your values, even if anxiety is present.
- Duration: Typically short-term, with sessions lasting around 8-12 weeks.

Psychodynamic Therapy:

Psychodynamic therapy is a longer-term therapeutic approach that delves into unconscious thoughts and early life experiences that may contribute to anxiety. It aims to uncover the root causes of emotional distress and anxiety.

- What to Expect: In psychodynamic therapy, you will explore past experiences and relationships to gain insights into how they may be affecting your present thoughts and behaviors. It's a more introspective form of therapy and can take longer to see results.
- Duration: Psychodynamic therapy can be long-term, with weekly sessions over months or even years.

3. The Therapist-Client Relationship

A key aspect of therapy is the relationship between you and your therapist. This therapeutic alliance plays a crucial role in your progress, as it creates a safe and supportive space where you can explore your feelings, share vulnerable experiences, and receive guidance.

What to Expect:

- Confidentiality: Therapy is a confidential space where you can speak openly about your thoughts, feelings, and experiences without fear of judgment. Your therapist is bound by ethical guidelines to keep what you discuss private (with a few exceptions, such as if you're at risk of harm).
- Respect and Understanding: A good therapist will treat you with empathy, respect, and nonjudgmental acceptance. They will listen actively and help you explore your emotions in a compassionate manner.
- Collaboration: Therapy is a collaborative process where you and your therapist work together to develop strategies and solutions to manage your anxiety. The therapist will guide you, but you will be an active participant in your own healing.

4. What to Expect from Sessions:

Therapy sessions typically last between 45 to 60 minutes, although the duration can vary. During the session, your therapist will help guide the conversation, but you will also have the opportunity to express how you're feeling, what challenges you're facing, and any progress you've made.

What to Expect:

- Regular Check-ins: Your therapist will likely ask about your current mood and any anxiety triggers you've encountered during the week. They may also inquire about how you've been applying techniques learned in therapy to real-life situations.
- Homework Assignments: In therapies like CBT, you may be given assignments or tasks to complete between sessions. These could include journaling, practicing relaxation techniques, or challenging negative thoughts.
- Emotional Processing: Sessions may involve processing difficult emotions or past experiences that are contributing to your anxiety. Your therapist will create a safe environment for you to explore and work through these emotions.

5. Duration and Frequency of Therapy

The frequency and duration of therapy vary depending on the type of therapy being used, your individual needs, and how well you respond to treatment. Some individuals may benefit from just a few sessions, while others may find that ongoing therapy provides continued support.

What to Expect:

- Short-Term Therapy: Many individuals with anxiety find relief in as little as 12-20 sessions, especially if they are utilizing CBT or other structured therapies.
- Long-Term Therapy: For individuals dealing with chronic anxiety or more complex underlying issues, long-term therapy may be necessary. In such cases, therapy may last for several months or even years.
- Session Frequency: Initially, therapy sessions may occur weekly, but they may become less frequent over time as you progress.

6. Tracking Progress in Therapy

One of the most important aspects of therapy is tracking your progress. As you work through your anxiety, you'll begin to notice changes in how you think, feel, and behave. These changes may take time, but with persistence, therapy can lead to lasting improvements in your mental health.

What to Expect:

- Self-Reflection: Your therapist may ask you to reflect on your progress and how your anxiety has changed since beginning therapy. They may also help you identify areas where you still struggle, allowing you to focus on those issues in subsequent sessions.
- Ongoing Adjustments: As you progress in therapy, your therapist may adjust the techniques or focus areas based on your evolving needs.

Therapy as a Path to Healing

Therapy is a highly effective and valuable tool for managing anxiety. By working with a therapist, you can gain insight into the causes of your anxiety, learn coping strategies, and develop healthier ways of thinking and behaving. Although the process may take time and effort, therapy offers the opportunity for long-term healing, personal growth, and improved mental well-being.

The therapeutic journey is deeply personal and unique to each individual, but with the right approach, commitment, and support, it can help you take meaningful steps toward managing your anxiety and living a more fulfilling life.

Chapter 11: Long-Term Strategies

Long-Term Strategies for Overcoming Anxiety and Panic Disorder

While immediate relief techniques such as deep breathing or grounding exercises are essential for managing acute anxiety and panic attacks, long-term strategies focus on creating lasting changes in how you think, respond, and manage stress in all aspects of your life. The journey to overcoming anxiety and panic disorder is not about eliminating anxiety entirely but learning to cope with it in a healthy way, reducing its impact, and empowering yourself to navigate life's challenges with greater ease.

In this chapter, we will explore long-term strategies for overcoming anxiety, addressing panic disorder, and developing skills to maintain calmness in both stressful and non-stressful situations. These strategies involve building resilience, changing thought patterns, making lifestyle changes, and creating a support system that reinforces your well-being.

The Power of Consistent Practice

One of the key components of long-term success in managing anxiety is consistent practice. Overcoming anxiety and panic disorder isn't a quick fix—it requires dedication, persistence, and the willingness to implement new habits and techniques over time. By making small but steady changes, you can significantly reduce the frequency and intensity of anxiety attacks and regain control over your life.

1. Building Resilience Over Time

Resilience is the ability to bounce back from setbacks and maintain a sense of inner strength, no matter the circumstances. When it comes to anxiety, resilience allows you to face anxiety-provoking situations without letting them overwhelm you. Building resilience involves developing mental toughness, emotional regulation, and a sense of self-efficacy—the belief that you have the skills to manage challenges.

What to Expect:

- Learning from Setbacks: When anxiety or panic strikes, it's essential to see these moments not as failures but as opportunities for growth. Each time you face an anxiety-inducing situation and manage to cope, you're strengthening your ability to handle similar situations in the future.
- Reframing Failures: Practice reframing setbacks as learning experiences. Instead of feeling discouraged by a panic attack or anxious moment, focus on what went well and what could be improved for next time. This mindset helps you approach your anxiety with a sense of curiosity rather than fear.

- Building Confidence: As you repeatedly apply coping strategies and see positive results, your confidence in managing anxiety will increase, making it easier to face future challenges.

2. Challenging Cognitive Patterns for Long-Term Relief

Long-term success in managing anxiety relies heavily on the ability to challenge and change the distorted thought patterns that fuel anxiety. Cognitive Behavioral Therapy (CBT) and other approaches such as Acceptance and Commitment Therapy (ACT) are powerful tools in helping individuals recognize their automatic, irrational thoughts and replace them with more balanced, realistic perspectives.

What to Expect:

- Identifying Cognitive Distortions: Over time, you will become more aware of the common cognitive distortions that trigger your anxiety, such as catastrophizing (expecting the worst) or overgeneralizing (thinking one mistake defines you). Recognizing these patterns is the first step toward changing them.
- Reframing Thoughts: With regular practice, you will become skilled at replacing negative or irrational thoughts with more helpful ones. For example, instead of thinking, "I can't handle this," you can reframe it to, "This situation is challenging, but I have the tools to manage it."

- Developing a Growth Mindset: Adopting a mindset that views challenges as opportunities for growth can reduce anxiety's grip on your life. Over time, you'll see anxiety as a manageable aspect of your experience, rather than something that controls you.

3. Practicing Mindfulness for Ongoing Calm

Mindfulness practices are key to managing anxiety over the long term. Learning to stay present, observe your thoughts without judgment, and remain calm in the face of anxiety can reduce the intensity of anxious feelings and create a sense of control. Mindfulness is not just about reducing anxiety; it's about developing a deep awareness of your thoughts, feelings, and physical sensations to prevent anxiety from taking over.

What to Expect:

- Mindfulness Meditation: Incorporating daily mindfulness meditation can train your mind to stay present, reducing the tendency to ruminate about past or future events. Even just 10 minutes a day can make a significant difference in managing anxiety.
- Mindful Breathing: Focusing on your breath throughout the day, especially during moments of anxiety, can help calm your nervous system and bring your attention back to the present moment.

- Mindful Awareness in Daily Activities: By practicing mindfulness during everyday tasks—like eating, walking, or washing dishes—you can strengthen your ability to remain calm and centered in both stressful and non-stressful situations.

4. Creating a Lifestyle that Supports Mental Health

A healthy lifestyle plays a pivotal role in reducing anxiety and improving overall mental well-being. By making intentional choices in areas like exercise, nutrition, sleep, and social support, you can build a foundation that supports long-term mental health and resilience.

What to Expect:

- Regular Exercise: Physical activity helps regulate stress hormones, release endorphins (the body's natural mood boosters), and improve sleep—all of which can reduce anxiety. Aim for activities that you enjoy, whether it's walking, yoga, swimming, or dancing.
- Balanced Nutrition: A nutrient-rich diet can have a positive impact on your mental health. Foods rich in omega-3 fatty acids, magnesium, and B-vitamins, along with limiting caffeine and sugar, can help stabilize your mood and reduce anxiety.
- Prioritizing Sleep: Sleep is essential for emotional regulation and overall well-being. Create a sleep routine

that supports restorative rest, aiming for 7-9 hours of quality sleep each night.
- Stress Management: Incorporating relaxation techniques into your daily life—such as deep breathing, progressive muscle relaxation, or guided imagery—can reduce the impact of daily stressors on your anxiety levels.

5. Cultivating Support and Connection

One of the most important long-term strategies for overcoming anxiety is to surround yourself with a supportive network of friends, family, and professionals. Having people to lean on can provide emotional support, reduce feelings of isolation, and remind you that you are not alone in your journey.

What to Expect:

- Building Strong Relationships: Cultivating meaningful relationships where you feel safe to express your feelings and challenges can create a sense of belonging and reduce anxiety. Communication and trust are key in these relationships.
- Engaging in Support Groups: Joining a support group for anxiety or panic disorder can help you connect with others who are experiencing similar challenges. It can be comforting and empowering to share your story, hear others' experiences, and gain new coping strategies.

- Professional Support: Therapy doesn't have to end once you start feeling better. Continuing to work with a therapist, even periodically, can provide ongoing support and ensure that you stay on track with your long-term mental health goals.

6. Developing Healthy Coping Strategies for Stressful Situations

As you progress in managing your anxiety, it's important to develop strategies that help you stay calm during stressful situations. Whether it's an upcoming presentation, a difficult conversation, or an unexpected event, having a set of tools to draw upon can help you feel more in control and less anxious.

What to Expect:

- Planning Ahead: Anticipating stressful situations and planning for how you will manage them can help reduce anxiety. For example, if you know you'll be in a crowded environment, practice grounding techniques or breathing exercises before you arrive.
- Staying Present in the Moment: Using mindfulness techniques to stay present can prevent your mind from spiraling into anxious thoughts about the future.
- Positive Self-Talk: Replace self-critical thoughts with affirmations and self-encouragement. Remind yourself of your strength, progress, and ability to manage stress.

- Relaxation Techniques: Keep relaxation strategies (like deep breathing, meditation, or visualization) readily available so you can use them when anxiety arises. These tools can help quickly shift your focus and calm your body and mind.

Embracing a Lifelong Journey of Mental Health

Long-term strategies for overcoming anxiety and panic disorder are about more than just managing symptoms; they're about creating lasting, positive changes in your mental, emotional, and physical health. Through consistent practice, building resilience, challenging negative thought patterns, and fostering healthy lifestyle choices, you can reduce the impact of anxiety on your life.

Remember, anxiety doesn't define you. It is something you can learn to manage, and through perseverance, support, and the right strategies, you can continue to thrive in the face of challenges. This journey is a lifelong process, but with the right tools and mindset, you can find peace, stability, and a greater sense of control over your anxiety and your life.

Developing a Personal Action Plan for Long-Term Anxiety Management

Creating a personal action plan is an essential part of maintaining long-term progress in managing anxiety and panic disorder. An action plan helps you structure your approach to mental health, providing clear goals, strategies, and techniques to navigate your journey. By breaking down your path into manageable steps, you empower yourself to take control of your anxiety and actively work toward reducing its impact on your life.

In this section, we will explore how to create an action plan that is tailored to your needs, strengths, and challenges. This plan should be flexible, allowing for adjustments as you progress, but it will serve as a roadmap for maintaining long-term mental health.

1. Assessing Your Current Situation

Before you begin developing an action plan, it's important to assess where you currently stand with your anxiety and panic disorder. This means taking stock of your symptoms, challenges, and triggers, as well as the coping strategies you have already tried. Being honest with yourself about where you are will help you identify areas that need the most attention and ensure that your action plan is both realistic and achievable.

Steps to Assess Your Situation:

- **Track Your Symptoms:** Keep a daily journal or use a mood-tracking app to monitor the frequency and intensity

of your anxiety symptoms. Note any patterns or triggers that seem to exacerbate your anxiety.
- **Identify Current Coping Mechanisms:** Take note of the techniques and strategies you currently use to manage anxiety (e.g., breathing exercises, mindfulness, therapy). Are they effective? Are there areas where you struggle to apply them?
- **Evaluate Your Support System:** Reflect on your current support system. Do you feel supported by friends, family, or a therapist? Are there gaps in your support network that need to be addressed?
- **Recognize Lifestyle Factors:** Assess your lifestyle choices, such as your exercise routine, nutrition, sleep habits, and stress management techniques. Are there any areas that could be improved to support your mental health?

2. Setting Clear and Achievable Goals

Once you have a clearer understanding of where you are, the next step is to set specific, measurable, achievable, relevant, and time-bound (SMART) goals for your anxiety management. These goals should focus on both short-term and long-term outcomes, helping you stay motivated and measure progress along the way.

- **Short-Term Goal:** "Practice deep breathing exercises for 5 minutes every morning for the next two weeks to reduce overall anxiety levels."
- **Long-Term Goal:** "Engage in regular exercise (at least 30 minutes, 3 times a week) for the next 6 months to improve physical health and decrease anxiety."
- **Process Goal:** "Track and record my anxiety levels every day for the next month to identify any patterns or triggers that contribute to my stress."

Make sure that each goal is aligned with your overall aim of managing anxiety and improving your well-being. These goals should be achievable and not too overwhelming, as unrealistic goals can lead to frustration and burnout.

3. Developing Coping Strategies for Different Scenarios

One of the most important parts of your action plan is developing a set of coping strategies to handle both acute anxiety and ongoing anxiety management. These strategies should be personalized to your preferences and comfort level, including tools you can rely on in different situations—whether you're experiencing a panic attack, dealing with general anxiety, or facing a stressful situation.

- **Grounding Techniques:** Develop a list of grounding techniques (e.g., 5-4-3-2-1 technique) that you can use when you feel disconnected or overwhelmed.
- **Breathing Exercises:** Incorporate deep breathing techniques such as diaphragmatic breathing or box breathing to calm your nervous system in stressful moments.
- **Mindfulness and Meditation:** Set a goal to practice mindfulness daily, whether through formal meditation, mindful walking, or mindful breathing, to help stay in the present moment.
- **Cognitive Reframing:** Use cognitive behavioral strategies to challenge negative thoughts. For example, identify irrational thoughts, like "I won't be able to handle this," and replace them with more balanced, realistic thoughts like "I've dealt with difficult situations before, and I have the tools to handle this one too."
- **Positive Affirmations:** Create a list of affirmations or mantras that you can repeat to yourself when you feel anxious, such as "I am capable of handling this" or "This feeling is temporary, and I can manage it."

4. Implementing Lifestyle Changes

Long-term anxiety management also requires adopting a lifestyle that supports mental and physical well-being. In your action plan, set specific goals for improving your overall health, as these changes can help reduce anxiety and improve your resilience.

Key Areas for Lifestyle Changes:

- **Exercise:** Schedule regular physical activity that you enjoy, such as walking, yoga, swimming, or cycling. Exercise releases endorphins, which can reduce anxiety and improve mood.
- **Nutrition:** Focus on eating a balanced diet rich in nutrients. Prioritize foods that support brain health and mood stability, such as leafy greens, fatty fish, and whole grains, while minimizing caffeine and sugar.
- **Sleep Hygiene:** Create a sleep routine to ensure you get adequate rest. Avoid screens before bedtime, establish a consistent sleep schedule, and create a calming environment for restful sleep.
- **Relaxation Techniques:** Incorporate relaxation practices such as progressive muscle relaxation (PMR), guided imagery, or self-hypnosis to reduce tension and anxiety throughout the day.

5. Building and Maintaining a Support System

Having a strong support system is essential in overcoming anxiety in the long run. A supportive network of friends, family, or professionals can provide emotional stability, reduce isolation, and offer a sounding board when you need it most.

Make a plan for how you can build or strengthen your support system to ensure you're not facing anxiety alone.

Support System Actions:

- **Therapy or Counseling:** If you're not already in therapy, include this as part of your action plan. Therapy, such as Cognitive Behavioral Therapy (CBT) or Acceptance and Commitment Therapy (ACT), can provide you with tools and strategies to better manage anxiety.
- **Support Groups:** Look for local or online support groups for individuals with anxiety or panic disorders. Sharing experiences and learning from others who are going through similar struggles can offer validation and encouragement.
- **Friends and Family:** Strengthen relationships with people who understand and support your journey. Practice open communication with those you trust, sharing your progress and struggles in an honest and vulnerable way.

6. Monitoring Progress and Adjusting the Plan

Your action plan should be a living document that evolves with your progress. Regularly assess how your coping strategies are working and if your goals need to be adjusted. Celebrate small victories along the way to stay motivated and remind yourself of how far you've come.

Steps to Monitor Progress:

- **Track Your Anxiety Levels:** Continue tracking your anxiety levels over time. Use tools like journaling or the Subjective Units of Distress (SUD) scale to assess changes and identify improvements.
- **Revisit Goals Regularly:** Set aside time each month to evaluate your progress toward your goals. Are you meeting your targets? What adjustments can you make to stay on track?
- **Celebrate Successes:** Recognize even small accomplishments. Whether it's a day with reduced anxiety or successfully using a coping technique in a stressful situation, celebrating progress reinforces your commitment to your mental health journey.

Staying Committed to Your Journey

Creating and following a personal action plan for managing anxiety is not a one-time effort but a continuous process. By setting clear goals, implementing coping strategies, and maintaining healthy lifestyle habits, you can build a solid foundation for long-term anxiety management. The key is to stay consistent, remain patient with yourself, and be adaptable as you move forward.

While setbacks are a natural part of any journey, your action plan equips you with the tools and strategies to overcome them. Over time, you will find yourself better equipped to handle stress, stay calm in challenging situations, and live a more balanced life free from the constant grip of anxiety.

Maintaining Progress and Celebrating Success

As you journey through overcoming anxiety and panic disorder, it's essential not only to focus on reaching your goals but also on maintaining the progress you've made. The road to mental well-being is ongoing, and while setbacks may occur, the goal is to create sustainable habits that continue to benefit you long after the initial phases of treatment. Recognizing your growth, staying committed to your strategies, and celebrating even small victories are vital to ensuring long-term success.

1. Reinforcing Positive Habits

One of the keys to maintaining progress is reinforcing the healthy habits you've developed over time. Anxiety management is about consistency, and the more regularly you engage in practices that support your mental and physical health, the more ingrained they will become. As you continue with your action plan, it's important to stay dedicated to the techniques that have proven most helpful and ensure they are a consistent part of your routine.

- **Make Anxiety Management a Daily Priority:** Incorporate the coping techniques, mindfulness exercises, and lifestyle changes that work best for you into your daily routine. Whether it's 10 minutes of meditation or regular physical activity, these small, consistent actions can build long-term resilience against anxiety.
- **Create a Routine:** Build structure into your day to help manage stress and anxiety. This could include setting regular sleep and exercise schedules, designating time for relaxation, or carving out space to practice mindfulness.
- **Review and Reflect:** Periodically review the coping strategies you've adopted. Are they still effective? Is there a new method or technique you'd like to try? Make adjustments as necessary to continue strengthening your mental health.

2. Overcoming Setbacks and Staying Resilient

It's important to understand that setbacks are a natural part of the recovery process. Anxiety may resurface at times, and panic attacks may still occur, even after periods of improvement. The key is to respond to these setbacks with resilience and self-compassion, rather than self-criticism. When you experience setbacks, it's not an indication that all progress has been lost; it's an opportunity to reinforce your coping skills and get back on track.

How to Handle Setbacks:

- **Accept the Experience:** Rather than seeing a setback as a failure, acknowledge it as a moment that doesn't define you or your progress. Everyone faces challenges, and it's how you respond that matters most.
- **Use the Setback as a Learning Opportunity:** Reflect on what may have triggered the setback. Did certain stressors or thoughts contribute? What tools or coping strategies can you use next time to prevent or minimize anxiety?
- **Practice Self-Compassion:** Be kind to yourself when setbacks occur. Remind yourself that recovery is a journey, and progress is measured by consistency over time, not perfection.

3. Tracking and Celebrating Successes

Celebrating even the smallest victories is a powerful way to maintain motivation and reinforce your efforts. Every moment you manage to reduce your anxiety, every coping strategy that works, and every day you feel calmer and more in control is a success. Acknowledging these moments helps you to recognize your strength and progress, even when the road feels long.

- **Create a Success Journal:** In addition to tracking your anxiety levels, keep a journal of your successes. Write down moments when you've used your coping strategies effectively, moments when anxiety didn't overwhelm you, or days when you felt more at ease. Reflecting on your wins can remind you of how much you've accomplished.
- **Reward Yourself:** Celebrate milestones by treating yourself. Whether it's indulging in a favorite hobby, enjoying a relaxing activity, or sharing your progress with a loved one, acknowledging your successes can reinforce positive behaviors.
- **Share with Supportive People:** Share your achievements with your support system—whether that's friends, family, or a therapist. Having others celebrate with you reinforces your journey and reminds you of the positive strides you've made.
- **Visual Reminders:** Consider creating a visual reminder of your progress, such as a progress chart or a gratitude board. Seeing your achievements over time can be motivating and help you stay focused on your long-term goals.

4. Staying Engaged in Your Mental Health Journey

Maintaining progress is also about staying engaged with your mental health journey. Even when you feel like your anxiety is under control, it's important to continue using your coping tools and engaging in practices that support your mental well-being. Staying proactive in your mental health ensures that you are equipped to handle stress and anxiety, both now and in the future.

How to Stay Engaged:

- **Continue Therapy or Counseling:** Even if you feel your anxiety has decreased, it can be helpful to continue with therapy, either on a regular or check-in basis. Therapy provides ongoing support, new tools, and strategies to maintain mental health.
- **Practice Mindfulness Regularly:** Incorporate mindfulness practices into your daily life, whether through meditation, mindful walking, or simple breathing exercises. The more you practice mindfulness, the easier it becomes to manage anxiety.
- **Join a Support Group:** Stay connected with others who are working through similar challenges by participating in support groups. Engaging with others provides encouragement, inspiration, and a reminder that you're not alone in your journey.
- **Refine Your Action Plan:** As you progress, revisit and update your personal action plan. Make adjustments based on what's working and what's not, and set new goals that reflect your current needs.

Remember that overcoming anxiety and panic disorder is a lifelong process. While the strategies and tools you've learned in this book can provide lasting relief, the journey doesn't end here. Embrace the ongoing nature of mental health care, and continue to evolve, learn, and adapt.

Life will always present new challenges and stressors, but with the right mindset and a solid set of coping strategies, you can approach these challenges with confidence and resilience. Your ability to manage anxiety is a testament to your strength and dedication to self-care.

Long-term anxiety management isn't about eliminating anxiety completely; it's about developing the skills to navigate it with ease and confidence. By maintaining progress, staying consistent with your coping techniques, and celebrating your successes, you'll continue to grow stronger and more resilient in the face of anxiety.

Over time, you'll find that your relationship with anxiety changes. What once felt overwhelming may eventually feel like just another part of your experience—something you can handle with calmness, grace, and perspective. By staying engaged with your mental health journey, you'll be empowered to thrive in both stressful and non-stressful situations, leading a life where anxiety no longer controls you but becomes a manageable aspect of your experience.

Hope for the Future: Shifting Perspectives and Creating a Positive Outlook

One of the most empowering aspects of managing anxiety is understanding that anxiety, in many ways, is a distortion of the future. As Martin Seligman, a leading figure in the field of positive psychology, has suggested, anxiety is often a "deformation" of what is yet to come. We are wired to imagine worst-case scenarios, to mentally prepare for potential threats, and to assume that the future will be filled with fear and danger. However, this mental distortion can hold us back from living fully in the present and rob us of the hope that things can get better.

By reframing our thoughts and challenging these distorted views of the future, we can break free from the grip of anxiety and cultivate a healthier, more optimistic outlook on life. This shift in perspective is not only about learning to manage anxiety, but also about creating a positive and realistic vision for the future—one that embraces the possibility of growth, resilience, and peace.

1. Recognizing Anxiety as a Deformation of the Future

Anxiety often involves imagining catastrophic outcomes that are highly unlikely to occur. We may overestimate the threat of a situation or feel paralyzed by fear of what might happen. This type of thinking—rooted in anticipation—turns potential future scenarios into sources of dread and worry. But the future, by nature, is unknown and uncontrollable, and the constant imagining of negative outcomes is a cognitive distortion.

How Anxiety Distorts the Future:

- **Catastrophic Thinking:** You may find yourself expecting the worst-case scenario to unfold, even when there is little evidence to support it. For example, before a presentation, you may believe that everything will go wrong and that you will be judged harshly.
- **Overestimating Danger:** Anxiety often exaggerates the level of threat in situations. A simple interaction, like meeting someone new, may feel like a life-or-death experience, though the actual risk is minimal.
- **Time Deformation:** Anxiety can cause you to feel like the future is always just around the corner, and it's filled with peril. This mindset frames a sense of urgency, as though there's no time to prepare or no way to escape.

By recognizing that anxiety often arises from this "distorted" vision of the future, we can begin to challenge it. The first step toward healing is understanding that the future has not happened yet, and that imagining it through the lens of anxiety only prevents us from fully experiencing the present moment.

2. Shifting Your Perspective: From Fear to Hope

In order to create a positive future, it's essential to shift from a mindset of fear and dread to one of hope and possibility. This involves intentionally training your mind to consider more realistic outcomes, to embrace uncertainty, and to view challenges as opportunities for growth rather than threats.

- **Focus on What You Can Control:** While the future will always be uncertain, there are aspects you can control—your actions, your responses, and your attitude. By focusing on the present moment and taking small, positive steps, you can feel more empowered and less overwhelmed by what lies ahead.
- **Challenge Catastrophic Thinking:** When you catch yourself imagining the worst, ask yourself: "What is the evidence that this outcome will happen?" Try to balance your thoughts by considering more likely, positive, or neutral possibilities. Use cognitive reframing techniques to remind yourself that not everything will go wrong.
- **Embrace Uncertainty:** One of the most difficult aspects of anxiety is the need for certainty. Learning to embrace uncertainty—rather than fearing it—can help you develop resilience. Understand that it's okay not to have all the answers or to know exactly what the future holds. Trust that you have the tools and the strength to navigate whatever comes your way.

- **Cultivate Optimism:** Positive psychology encourages the practice of optimism—not as a denial of life's challenges but as a choice to focus on the positive aspects of your life and the future. Try to visualize positive outcomes for situations that make you anxious. Remind yourself of your strengths and past successes, and believe in your ability to cope with challenges.

3. Creating a New, Positive Narrative

As you work through the process of managing anxiety, it becomes important to rewrite the narrative you tell yourself about the future. The stories we tell ourselves about what will happen are incredibly powerful, and they shape our emotional and physical responses. Shifting this narrative to one that is more hopeful, empowering, and focused on possibilities can help reduce anxiety and foster a sense of peace.

Steps to Create a Positive Narrative:

- **Reframe Your Fears:** Instead of focusing on potential negative outcomes, reframe your fears into challenges that you can handle. For example, instead of thinking, "I'm going to fail and everyone will judge me," you might reframe it as, "This is an opportunity to learn and grow, and even if things don't go perfectly, I will handle it and learn from the experience."
- **Focus on Strengths:** Reflect on the strengths that have helped you through difficult situations in the past. Remind yourself of the resources, both internal (like resilience,

perseverance, and emotional intelligence) and external (like support from loved ones, therapy, and coping skills), that you have at your disposal.
- **Visualize Positive Outcomes:** Visualization is a powerful tool that can help you focus on positive possibilities rather than worst-case scenarios. Before a potentially anxiety-provoking event, take a few minutes to imagine it going well. See yourself succeeding or handling the situation with calm and confidence. Visualizing success can help you feel more prepared and reduce anxiety about the future.

4. Embracing the Present Moment for a Brighter Future

While shifting your perspective on the future is important, it is equally essential to remain grounded in the present moment. Anxiety often stems from ruminating about what could happen, what might go wrong, or what is out of our control. Focusing on the present moment, practicing mindfulness, and letting go of the need to predict the future can significantly reduce anxiety.

How to Stay Present:

- **Practice Mindfulness:** Engage in mindfulness exercises, such as deep breathing, meditation, or mindful observation. By focusing on your breath, your body, or the environment around you, you can bring yourself back

to the present moment and interrupt the cycle of anxious thoughts about the future.
- **Cultivate Gratitude:** Develop a gratitude practice by writing down or mentally noting things you are thankful for each day. Gratitude helps you shift your focus from anxiety-inducing thoughts to positive aspects of your life, reinforcing a sense of abundance and well-being.
- **Engage in Activities That Ground You:** Engage in activities that pull you into the present moment, such as exercise, hobbies, or spending time with loved ones. These activities can help you stay focused on what's happening right now rather than worrying about what's ahead.

5. Hope for the Future: A Life Beyond Anxiety

The most powerful tool in overcoming anxiety is hope. Hope for the future is not about ignoring the challenges you may face, but about trusting that, no matter what happens, you are capable of handling it. By creating a new, positive perspective, you can reshape the way you view both the present and the future. Anxiety may still arise, but with these tools and strategies, it no longer has to dominate your life or control your thoughts.

Anxiety's distortion of the future can feel overwhelming and isolating, but by shifting your perspective and creating a new narrative, you can break free from its grip. The future is not determined by your anxious thoughts, but by the actions you take today. By adopting a more positive, hopeful outlook, embracing uncertainty, and focusing on the present moment, you can build a future that is full of possibility, resilience, and peace.

The key is to remember: anxiety does not define you, and the future is not set in stone. With the right mindset, coping strategies, and support, you have the power to shape your future in a way that aligns with your values, hopes, and aspirations.

he Power of the Present: Finding Calmness in the Now

As we navigate the complexities of anxiety and mental health, it's essential to understand how our relationship with time—both the past and the future—affects our emotional state. Often, our anxieties arise from the mental patterns we develop around these two dimensions of time: the past and the future. The past can pull us into depression, while the future can keep us locked in anxiety, but the true state of calmness resides in the present moment.

The Past and Depression:

The past is a common source of depression. When we dwell on past mistakes, regrets, or painful experiences, we can become trapped in negative cycles of rumination. The mind replays old events over and over, often exaggerating their impact or distorting their significance, creating a mental environment where it becomes difficult to move forward.

- **Rumination:** When we focus on what has already happened, we can get stuck in patterns of overthinking, reliving past failures, or dwelling on old wounds. This type of rumination prevents us from healing because it keeps us mentally anchored in a time that is no longer present.
- **Regret and Shame:** The feeling of regret about what we could have done differently, or the shame of mistakes made, can prevent us from accepting what happened and moving forward. We can become so consumed by the past that it clouds our ability to fully engage with the present moment.

In many ways, depression can be seen as an emotional response to the past. It is our mind's way of holding onto negative experiences, often turning them into lasting emotional scars. However, by learning to let go of the past and focus on the present, we can begin to free ourselves from the weight of these emotional burdens.

The Future and Anxiety:

On the other hand, the future is the breeding ground for anxiety. Our minds often jump ahead, imagining all the possible negative outcomes, often without any solid evidence. The fear of what might happen—or the anticipation of potential failure—can cause an overwhelming sense of dread, leaving us feeling anxious, nervous, or even paralyzed by the uncertainty that the future represents.

- **Catastrophic Thinking:** This is the tendency to imagine the worst-case scenario. Anxiety thrives on uncertainty, and the human brain can easily amplify fears about the future, creating a narrative that is far more dramatic and improbable than the reality.
- **Lack of Control:** We cannot predict the future, and that lack of control can feel unsettling. Anxiety often stems from this unknown—fearing what will happen next, whether we'll be ready for it, or how we might cope with it.
- **Future-Oriented Rumination:** Much like rumination about the past, future-oriented rumination keeps us stuck in a loop of worry. We constantly question "What if?" scenarios, imagining every possible way things could go wrong.

Living in a constant state of worry about the future can prevent us from fully experiencing the present. When we focus on future uncertainties, we miss out on the richness of life as it unfolds in the here and now.

The True Calmness: The Present Moment

The only true state of calmness we can experience is in the present moment. It's only in the present that we can engage with life directly, make decisions, and take action. When we are mindful of the present, we move beyond the constraints of our anxiety and depression, finding peace in the act of simply *being*.

In the present moment, there is no worry about what could have been or what might be. There is only *what is*. This state of mindfulness is where we can find true peace—free from the weight of past regrets and future fears.

Why the Present Moment Is Where Calmness Resides:

- **Mindfulness:** Mindfulness is the practice of being fully present and aware of our thoughts, feelings, and environment in the here and now, without judgment. It allows us to step outside of our worries about the future or our regrets about the past and connect with our immediate experience.

- **Acceptance of the Moment:** In the present, we can accept things as they are—without the need to change them or worry about what's coming next. By cultivating an attitude of acceptance, we can decrease stress and anxiety.
- **Control and Empowerment:** The present is the only time we can control. We cannot change what happened in the past, and we cannot predict what will happen in the future. But in the present, we can take meaningful actions, practice self-care, and make choices that benefit our mental health.

When we ground ourselves in the present moment, we take back control of our emotional state. We step out of the patterns of anxiety and depression that are tied to past and future concerns, and instead, we place our focus on what we can do *now*—to nurture ourselves, to address challenges, and to foster a sense of peace and stability.

The Power of the Now: Living with Purpose

When we shift our focus from the past and future to the present, we open ourselves up to new possibilities. The present moment is where we can create meaning and purpose, where we can connect with others, and where we can find true joy and peace. It's the space where we have the most agency and the power to create positive changes in our lives.

Practical Steps to Stay Present:

- **Practice Grounding Techniques:** Grounding exercises, like the 5-4-3-2-1 technique, can help you refocus on the present by engaging your senses and drawing your attention away from anxious thoughts. By identifying five things you can see, four things you can touch, three things you can hear, two things you can smell, and one thing you can taste, you bring yourself back to the here and now.
- **Mindful Breathing:** Simple breathing exercises, like inhaling deeply for four counts, holding for four counts, and exhaling for four counts, can calm your nervous system and anchor you in the present moment.
- **Engage in Activities You Enjoy:** Whether it's painting, hiking, reading, or spending time with loved ones, engaging in activities that bring you joy can help you remain focused on the present, allowing you to experience life as it unfolds.
- **Use Self-Talk to Reframe:** When you catch yourself ruminating on the past or worrying about the future, use positive self-talk to bring yourself back to the present. Remind yourself that you can handle things as they come and that your anxiety does not need to control your experience.

Conclusion: Embracing the Present for True Calmness

Anxiety and depression often arise from the mental habits we develop around the past and the future. The past can trap us in regret and sadness, while the future can feed our fears and uncertainties. But the key to overcoming these mental patterns lies in cultivating a strong connection to the present moment.

By practicing mindfulness and focusing on what we can do right now, we open ourselves up to peace and calmness. The future is uncertain, and the past is gone, but the present is where we can find true control, purpose, and joy. By learning to stay grounded in the now, we empower ourselves to live with less anxiety and more peace.

So, the next time you feel overwhelmed by what's coming or what's already happened, remember: the present moment is the only place where true calmness resides. Step into the now, and reclaim your peace.

Embracing Life Beyond Anxiety: Forgetting About Anxiety, Saving the Fear for Tomorrow

One of the most liberating steps in overcoming anxiety is realizing that *you do not have to live with it all the time.* Anxiety, while a natural response to stress, does not have to define who you are or dictate how you experience life. It can feel consuming at times, but with the right strategies and mindset, you can learn to manage it—and eventually, leave it behind.

The concept of *forgetting about anxiety* may sound radical, but it is possible. Anxiety thrives when we focus on it, give it our attention, and let it dictate how we respond to life. However, by developing healthier thought patterns, using mindfulness techniques, and embracing the present moment, we can distance ourselves from the grip of anxiety. The key is to accept that anxiety is just a temporary feeling, not a permanent part of who we are.

Saving the Fear for Tomorrow or Never:

One powerful approach to managing anxiety is realizing that fear is often something reserved for *tomorrow, next week or next year*, not today. Anxiety frequently lingers in anticipation of events that haven't even happened yet. When you catch yourself in anxious thinking, remind yourself that the fear can be put on hold. It's not useful to borrow stress from the future. In fact, by doing so, you're depriving yourself of the ability to truly live in the present.

You don't need to carry tomorrow's worries today. When you begin to consciously separate fear from your current reality, you free yourself from the constant cycle of anxiety. This approach requires practice, but over time, you'll notice a profound shift in your emotional landscape. You'll start to recognize the space between your present self and your anxious thoughts about the future.

Final Thoughts and Encouragement:

If you're struggling with anxiety right now, know that it doesn't have to control your life forever. Every step you take toward understanding and managing your anxiety is a victory. Recovery is not about eliminating anxiety completely, but rather about finding a balance where it no longer dominates your thoughts or decisions.

- **You Are Not Alone:** Anxiety is one of the most common mental health challenges people face, and you don't have to go through it alone. Whether through therapy, support groups, or confiding in loved ones, there are resources and people who understand what you're going through and can help guide you.
- **It Takes Time:** Change doesn't happen overnight. Anxiety, like any emotional challenge, takes time to understand, manage, and eventually overcome. Be patient with yourself and recognize each small victory along the way. Progress may be slow, but it is real.
- **Your Journey is Unique:** Your path to overcoming anxiety will be uniquely yours. It may take time to discover what works best for you—whether that's therapy, medication, mindfulness, or lifestyle changes. Trust that the process is as individual as you are. There is no one-size-fits-all solution, but there is a solution that fits you.
- **Celebrate Your Strengths:** Every moment you face your anxiety and choose to move forward is a testament to your strength and resilience. It takes courage to confront

fears, break patterns, and work toward healing. You are stronger than you may realize.
- **Hope for the Future:** The future holds limitless possibilities. As you move beyond anxiety, you open yourself up to a life filled with joy, peace, and fulfillment. Anxiety may still show up now and then, but with the right tools, mindset, and support, you will always have the ability to reclaim your calmness and move forward with strength.

In Conclusion:

Anxiety does not define you, nor does it have to limit your potential. By embracing life beyond anxiety, you allow yourself to live with more freedom, peace, and joy. The fear you carry about the future can be saved for tomorrow, while today can be about embracing the present moment and the calmness it offers. Remember, you have everything you need to move through this—and you have the ability to thrive.

So, take a deep breath. Let go of the worry about the future. Know that you are enough, just as you are. Take it one step at a time, and always believe that peace is possible. You are on your way to a brighter, calmer tomorrow. I hope this book will help you to cultivate a calm mindset so that you can be the best version of yourself and beyond!

Made in the USA
Monee, IL
05 January 2025